The Milk Book

THE MILK OF HUMAN KINDNESS IS NOT PASTEURIZED...

"How Science Is Destroying Nature's Nearly Perfect Food."

By **William Campbell Douglass II**, MD

This publication is designed to provide accurate and authoritative information in regard to the subject matter covered. It is sold with the understanding that the publisher is not engaged in rendering medical, or other professional service. If medical advice or other expert assistance is required, the services of a competent professional person should be sought. This book is not a substitute for medical advice.

Rhino Publishing, S.A.

The Milk Book

THE MILK OF HUMAN KINDNESS
IS NOT PASTEURIZED...

"How Science Is Destroying Nature's Nearly Perfect Food."

Copyright © 1984, 1995, 2003
by
William Campbell Douglass II, MD

All rights reserved. This book, or parts thereof, may not be reproduced in any form without permission from the publisher or the author; exceptions are made for brief excerpts or quotations used in published reviews or articles.

ISBN 9962-636-54-X

Cover illustration by
Alex Manyoma (alex@3dcity.com)

Please, visit Rhino's website for other publications from
Dr. William Campbell Douglass
www.rhinopublish.com

Dr. Douglass' "Real Health" alternative medical newsletter
is available at www.realhealthnews.com

RHINO PUBLISHING, S.A.
World Trade Center
Panama, Republic of Panama

Voicemail/Fax
International: + 416-352-5126
North America: 888-317-6767

DEDICATION

to Jack Mathis

CONTENTS

ACKNOWLEDGEMENTS

Dr. H. Leon Abrams, Jr. for unselfishly opening his files to me.

Jack Mathis, without whose help this book could not have been written.

Harold Steuve, the Steuve family and the staff of Alta-Dena Dairy for their help and inspiration.

Paul Virgin of the Alta-Dena Dairy for his time and advice.

Dee Cochran for typing the manuscript from my illegible writing.

Dr. Derrick B. Jelliffee for allowing me to quote from his landmark work *Human Milk in the Modern World.*

Dr. Paul Fleiss, a pediatrician ahead of his time, for his assistance.

Dr. Robert Mendelsohn, my fearless leader in the movement to resist the homogenization of American medicine.

Dr. Robert Pottenger, of the Price-Pottenger Foundation, for allowing me access to the *History of Randleigh Farms.*

Ed O'Neal for his patience and hard work.

Hugh Allen for his bright idea.

Col. McCrary for his generosity.

Al Mason and Virginia Wilder for cleaning up my grammar.

PREFACE

Don't skim over this book about milk. The health and wealth of this nation are inextricably tied into our agriculture. Our greatest agricultural loss today is due to our senseless destruction of fresh milk through pasteurization, ultra-pasteurization, and now ultra high temperature pasteurization which turns a great food into a white, "milkflavored drink," about as nutritious as milk of magnesia.

Don't skim over the footnotes either. If you do, you'll miss a lot of good stuff.*

With proper understanding of milk, and its destructive effects (when heat-treated) and the remarkable therapeutic effects when used raw, we can cut *billions of dollars* off our medical bills, make ourselves infinitely more healthy, and actually raise the I.Q. of our children. With smarter children we will add greatly to our scientific and cultural wealth. I do not consider it an exaggeration to say that the nation's destiny will be affected by what we do about milk. If you doubt this, read Chapter III first. This chapter should convince you that a switch to unprocessed, that is unpasteurized, milk should be a national priority.

If you listen to the advertising of the dairy industry, one gets the impression that milk is the perfectfood,and, if you don't stoke your children with at least a quart of milk a day (each), you are guilty of child abuse or at least neglect.

---

* Just testing you

On the other hand, some nutritionists, medical organizations, government agencies, and doctors warn of
the dangers of fat and cholesterol in milk and milk products. We are told that "Mr. Cholesterol" is going to get us
if we don't restrict our intake of dairy products, especially eggs, meat, and demon milk.

A small group of nutritionists are so anti-milk that
they state flatly: No one should drink milk after eighteen
months of age-period. This is the "milk is only for babies"
school of nutrition.

Another small but growing faction of nutritionists
says that the problem with milk is *American* milk. That is,
milk is okay when used the way nature made it, but it's
changed into a useless, and actually dangerous product
when processed by modern dairy methods. This group,
composed of some experienced nutritionists, presents
evidence that pasteurized, homogenized milk actually
causes the very disease it is supposed to help prevent -
tooth decay! They also point out that milk may cause arteriosclerosis and thus heart attack, not because of the fat
or cholesterol content, but because of the way the milk is
altered by the pasteurization and homogenization processes. They ask, "Is milk the perfect food, or is it, because
of modern processing methods, a major health hazard?"

There are advocates of goat milk, camel milk, yak
milk, mithan milk, skim milk, and the non-milk, soy
milk. One physician/nutritionist says the only way to
drink milk is to take pure cream and dilute it with water.

Milk is as American as Coca-Cola and at least half
the population drinks milk. Most of the rest ingest it in
one form or another - cheese, bakery goods, and in the
process of cooking in general. But is American processed
milk a nutritional stalwart that helps build strong bodies
and good teeth, or is it, like Coca-Cola, just another form
of junk food?

We will cover a vast array of subjects in this book such
as raw milk, medical milk therapy, human milk, margarine

and butter, the sudden infant death syndrome, and the great yogurt rip-off, but *the major thrust of this book will be to warn you of the dangers of pasteurized milk and to inform you about the incredible health benefits to be gained from drinking fresh, untreated, unpasteurized, in other words, raw milk.* We will attempt to convince you that raw certified milk will keep you free of disease, improve your sex life, give you more energy and stamina, and extend your life by at least ten years.

That's a big order. Read on—this book may change your life.

FOREWORD TO THE THIRD EDITION

Although written in 1984, *The Milk Book* is as timely today as ever. I wouldn't change a word of it. In fact, I'm not going to.

Only recently has science confirmed what we first said more than eight years ago in this book: Adding vitamin D to milk is a risky business. It is entirely unnecessary to "fortify" milk with this highly toxic substance.

Not too long ago, the *New England Journal of Medicine* reported eight cases of vitamin D intoxication resulting from excessive fortification of commercial milk. Symptoms included anorexia, weight loss, constipation, weakness, fatigue, inability to think correctly, and something they described as "failure to thrive." You wouldn't catch all that stuff from my Great-Grandma Bell's milk!

According to the article, the artificial baby formulas were even worse than dairy milk. *None* of the formulas tested had the amount of vitamin D stated on the label; almost all contained excessive amounts of this toxic vitamin.

The anti-cholesterol propaganda blitz has increased dramatically since this book was first published. Children are now being denied whole milk because pediatricians are obsessed with the cholesterol myth. These same gutless wonders don't say anything about children drinking half-a-dozen bottles of Coca-Cola a day, starting before breakfast. But kids can't get a decent glass of milk!

Even if Mom buys whole milk, thinking it is better for her growing child than that sickly blue stuff called skim, she can't win, because all of the commercial milk is homogenized. I'm convinced that homogenization is even *more* detrimental to the nutritional quality of milk than the heat processing called pasteurization. (See Chapter VII—"Udder Menace.")

Meat is in the doghouse and the animal rights movement has heated up to a point that we may all be forced to become vegetarians. If one of your friends (or children) has succumbed to the anti-meat hysteria, have him or her read Chapter XII— "Let 'Em Eat Steak."

And let me also put in a plug here for Chapter X, "This Greasy Counterfeit." It really infuriates me that you simply cannot find butter in a restaurant anymore; it's always some kind of "spread." (I guess they're ashamed to admit it's margarine.) For the full story of the shameful grease that is masquerading as God's butter, please read Chapter X.

The longest chapter in the book is the one on breast-feeding (Chapter IX—"Udder Perfection"). I am honored that my writings had at least a little influence, along with the work of the La Leche League and the efforts of my great good friend, Dr. Robert Mendelsohn, on the increase in breast-feeding in this country.

You might remember that this movement was met with stony silence by the pediatricians—until they realized they were looking pretty anti-nature and did a 180-degree turnaround. Now they claim credit for the revival!

But that battle also is not over. America's mothers are backsliding. The number of mothers breast-feeding is dropping precipitously, because it's not convenient or compatible with the image of the modern, liberated woman, I guess. The artificial-baby-formula companies are gearing up for another propaganda blitz against feeding au naturel. I've even seen articles questioning the safety or desirability of feeding babies natural breast milk! Can you believe that?

Most readers of this book have never seen, much less tasted, natural milk from a cow. I'm talking about the straight stuff, with the cream left where it belongs—on the top of the milk—and no vitamin D or other artificial elements added.

Once you have read The Milk Book, I hope you will want to drink only natural, unpasteurized, unhomogenized milk yourself. This is easier said than done. At the time of this writing, there is only one dairy in the entire United States producing unpasteurized, unhomogenized milk: Alta Dena Dairy in Chino, California. Sadly, their days appear to be numbered.

The media, in collusion with the dieticians, the American Heart Association, and the food industry, have done such a colossal job of indoctrinating the American people on the supposed dangers of cholesterol and the drinking of unpasteurized ("raw') milk that it is no longer available in most states.

What can you do? Let me suggest five things:

(1). Contact your state legislators and demand that they permit you the freedom to choose what sort of milk you will drink.

(2). Ditto your federal senators and representatives.

(3). Tell the PDA to stop acting like commissars and start acting like what they're supposed to be, public servants.

(4). Buy a cow and milk it yourself.

(5). If that's too much trouble, make friends with someone who owns a cow and come to some private arrangement with him/her.

In conclusion, let me note that writing *The Milk Book* was the most fun I have ever had with a typewriter. I am even more pleased with this book now, because it has endured the test of time. I hope you will agree—and will urge your own children to read it, too.

FOREWORD

This important book should be read by two groups of people—those who drink milk and those who don't. Both groups will learn that, "Is milk good or bad for you?" is the wrong question. The right question is, "What *kind* of milk should you drink?"

William Campbell Douglass, M.D., in his eminently readable and authoritatively documented book, teaches us a valuable lesson in semantics – the opposite of "dirty" is not "pasteurized" or "homogenized". The opposite of "dirty" is "clean".

And clean milk means raw certified milk!

Even more remarkable than the message of this book is the messenger. Douglass belongs to the profession of Modern Medicine, a group noted, over the past five decades, for its belief in "better living through chemistry."

Reared in a tradition that reveres the fluoridation of our water supplies and eagerly anticipates the irradiation of our food supplies, impeccably credentialed Dr. Douglass is practically unique in Modern Medicine in arguing for a clean milk supply.

Don't look for other MD's to join Bill Douglass' crusade against milk pollution. Habituated to creating mini-Love Canals in the blood streams of their private patients, modern physicians are unwilling to marshal the righteous indignation and careful reasoning necessary to protest against pollution of the public's water, food and milk.

Not only is Douglass' case against pasteurization and homogenization compelling, but this book helps clarify many other issues (vegetarianism vs. meat eating; the cholesterol controversy; goat's milk vs. cow's milk), and offers valuable insights into osteoporosis, tall stature of Americans, cancer, and vitamins. Bill Douglass' breezy style — complete with hilarious footnotes—adds the dimension of entertainment to a fine educational experience.

Robert S. Mendelsohn, M.D.
Author, "Confessions of a Medical Heretic"
August, 1984

INTRODUCTION

Factual and funny, witty and blisteringly honest... filled with truth and hilarity—all the stuff that usually only fiction is made of.

A vital food resource destroyed through greed, ignorance, vindictiveness and fanatical prejudice.

It is all here in this uncommonly readable book. The talented Dr. Douglass has described the destructive effects of pasteurization of milk and the utter ruthlessness and dishonesty of state government protecting a favored industry.

The story he tells of the State of California and its persecution of the Alta-Dena Dairies is unique in the annals of state government.

The battle is almost won—by the panzers of pasteurization. At the time of this writing, the federal government has moved in to crush Alta Dena and Mathis Dairies. A regulation is being proposed that will make the sale of raw milk illegal nationwide. The producers of fresh, clean milk will be classified with heroin, marijuana and cocaine peddlers, and, probably more severely dealt with.

The American Medical Association, the American Veterinary Association, all of the State health departments, the American Dietetic Association, the American Academy of Pediatrics, the milk lobby, and those consummate meddlers and anti-free enterprise fanatics, Ralph Nader and Dr. Sidney Wolf, are arrayed against the only two clean dairies left in the entire United States to the detriment of the well being and free choice of the people of America.

To the rescue, just in time, comes this factual, funny, first; the only publication in print that tells the true and complete story about milk. The book will probably be suppressed. You are unlikely to find it in your local bookstore. But, if a million copies of this book can be distributed, the battle for clean, fresh milk can still be won.

Buy this book by the case from the publisher. Give them to your friends and relatives for birthdays and Christmas (or Hannukkah, Bastille Day, Labor Day, Fourth of July, St. Patrick's Day, or National Pork Week). Send a copy to your representatives at the local, state and federal level. Send a copy to the President. If he receives a freight car load of them, maybe it will get his attention.

Time is running out. But, the war isn't over until it's over.

Clean, unprocessed milk is essential to health, especially for our children and the elderly. Only you, and tens of thousands of other caring Americans can save this vital food, this "life's blood" given by God to His children for vibrant good health.

Turn to the last page in the book for your ammunition. Order more copies than you can afford because you can't afford not to!

Maureen Kennedy Salaman
President, National Health Federation

Chapter I

YELLOW COWS
THE HISTORY OF MILK

One of the most revolutionary developments in human history was the invention of milking animals for food by the ancients of Southwestern Asia. It's hard to understand why no one else thought of it for hundreds of years. South American Indians had an ample supply of milk available in the llama but never took advantage of it. North American Indians had the buffalo, but she doesn't milk easily.* The Chinese and Japanese are pretty smart, but they didn't think of it either. Milking was introduced there only within the last century.

The goat was probably the first animal to have the honor of being milked. Horses were too big, dogs too small and cats wouldn't put up with it. But domesticated horses now produce great milk-better than cows. See Chapter XIII.

The earliest pictures of milking show the milker sitting directly *behind* the cow. Not a smart idea. Man learns everything the hard way. As milking caught on, the technique was extended to almost all domesticated animals except the pig.**

The revolutionary adoption of milking domesticated animals for human food enormously increased man's protein supply, and milk with grain became the standard diet of most of the world. Until very recently, the peasants of Scotland ate little else. Doctor Samuel Johnson made the comment that oats are food for horses in England and food for men in Scotland. To which the Scots replied, "And where else will you find such horses and such men?"

---

* Too omery.
** Did you every try to milk a pig?

When the English came to Jamestown in 1611, they brought their cows with them. One can imagine the astonishment of the Indians on first encountering these strange, docile, short-haired "buffalo". With the milk, they brought tuberculosis, brucellosis (undulant fever), typhoid, and other diseases the Indians didn't need. Don't misunderstand me. It wasn't the fault of the milk. It was diseased people who contaminated the milk that caused the problems. We'll explain that later.

During the Renaissance period, the farmers painted their cows yellow to stimulate milk production.* Cows and their cousins, such as the ox, have played an important role throughout history.** If you are really interested in the cow's point of view on history, religion, and the arts, read The Cow Book by Marc Gallant (Alfred A. Knopf, N.Y., 1983).***

Milk remained an honest product for over two hundred years. Sure, it was contaminated, but so was everything else. Then the first of the milk manipulators came along- Gale Borden. By condensing milk, Borden discovered that it would keep for longer periods due to its high sugar content. He patented the process and it has been downhill for milk ever since.

But the original culprit was probably the Italian biologist Lazzaro Spallangani who popularized the preserving of food through heating in 1765.

1873 was a fateful year for milk in the United States. Dr. Abraham Jacobi publicly urged the boiling or cooking of all milk used in infant feeding because of the frightful carnage of babies at that time from infectious diseases. At times the death toll reached the unbelievable figure of 65%, and the annual loss of babies throughout the country, largely due to unsanitary conditions with consequent fatal infections, exceeded 250,000.

---

* It didn't work.
** They did most of the heavy work.
*** It's a wondeerful book.

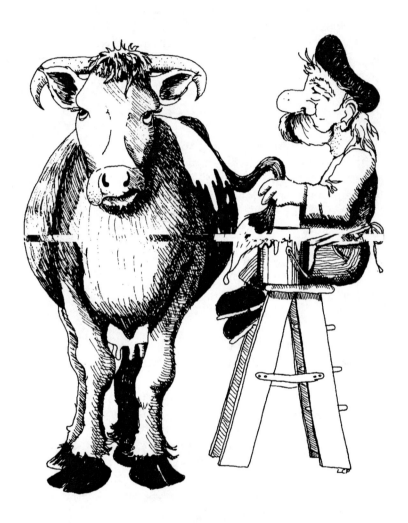

Painting Cows Yellow to Increase Milk Productions

Cows in the late 1800's were fed on garbage. The Commissioner of the New York State Health Department, Dr. Herman E. Hillaboe, reported that cows were milked in a mixture of manure and mud, dust, dirt, filth, and disease-germs were as much the total product that people drank as was the milk itself. On farms, pails that were used to carry slop to the pigs were also used to convey milk to human consumers.

The New York philanthropist, Nathan Straus, lost a child from contaminated milk (diphtheria). This prompted him to start his famous "milk stations" where only cooked (pasteurized) milk was supplied to the poor of the city. The effectiveness of heat-treated milk in reducing mortality in the late nineteenth and early twentieth centuries is indisputable. In a seven year period, starting in 1897, the death rate among children in New York City dropped from 42% to 22% with the only discernible change being the pasteurization, heat-treatment of milk.

The first successful Tuberculin test for dairy herds began in 1890. In 1893, under the direction of Dr. Henry L. Coit of Newark, New Jersey, there began a serious effort to control the cleanliness of milk. Dr. Coit deserves some sort of medal for his pioneer work in cleaning up the milk industry. This certification process was started in Essex County, New Jersey, rapidly spreading around the country, and in 1907 the certification of milk, the insuring by a group of concerned physicians that the milk was pure enough to drink, was generally standard.-

Pasteurization began in 1895, and thus began the unfortunate habit of not worrying about cleanliness in the dairy because, with the heating of milk, cleanliness was no longer considered necessary. The bacteria in the milk would simply be boiled, killing the germs, and then the milk could be sold in this adulterated form. It has been sold that way ever since, and, *because of pasteurization*, tuberculosis was not completely eliminated from cows in the United States until 1941. If the United States Public Health Service and the American Medical Association had done the responsible thing and backed the various medical milk commissions' efforts to keep milk clean, tuberculosis could have been eliminated from American cows many decades sooner.

Dr. Henry Coit, the father of certified milk, recognized clearly that top quality milk depended upon getting the milk fresh from the cow and not heating it as is done in the pasteurization process. He recognized that the best way to present the best and most nutritious product to the public was to deliver it as made by nature from a completely clean environment.

In 1891, Coit received an even stronger impetus to crusade for clean milk. His first son, only two years old, died from contaminated milk. It took six years for Dr. Coit to talk the first dairyman, Steven Francisco, into producing "certified milk." The term "certified" meant that the milk was inspected by a board of physicians and was certified by them to meet rigid standards of cleanliness.

By 1904, thirteen years after the tragic death of Coit's son, certified dairies were being inspected regularly. But these progressive dairies represented only a tiny percentage of milk production, and the battle for disease-free milk was only beginning. It was estimated in 1905 that 35% of the twenty-four million dairy cattle had tuberculosis and over 10% had brucellosis. Today's raw certified milk must not have a germ count higher than 10,000 per cubic centimeter. In 1911 the milk being served *in hospitals* often had a count as high as *twenty million* germs per cubic centimeter.

The Medical Milk Commission, the group of physicians that inspected and "certified" the raw milk as meeting the rigid standards of safety, grew rapidly across the country, and, by 1930, clean, unpasteurized, raw milk was generally available across the country.

If this healthy trend had continued, *pasteurized milk would have never been accepted by the American people.* Certification of raw milk by medical experts was rapidly eliminating the disease problem from milk. They had proven that tampering with milk by heat-treatment pasteurization was entirely unnecessary. The people did not trust pasteurization for many reasons, the main one being the nutrition factor. Hall and Trout, in their book *Milk Pasteurization*, admit that, due to the deep-seated distrust of pasteurization, "one is astounded that the process ever was successfully introduced." But the pasteurization fanatics were determined to eliminate raw milk from the dinner table. They had accepted pasteurization as a veritable religion, and, although the Medical Milk Commission had proven beyond a doubt that *clean milk*, not *heated* milk, was the answer to the problem, they moved forward with a relentless propaganda blitz. The devious war fought against raw certified milk will be discussed in detail in Chapters IV, V, and VI.

Human milk also has a long and interesting history. In Sparta, 400 B.C., it was decreed that mothers must breast feed their babies. The Koran dictates that, "mothers shall suckle their children for two years." Caesar ridiculed the mothers of Rome who retained wet nurses for their children. Early American Indians believed that the longer a child received breast milk, the longer it would live.* It was not uncommon for Indian "babies" to be suckled until the age of nine years. A half-century ago, Eskimos were known to nurse their babies up to 15 years.**

In the 18th century, there was a great faith in the healing and preventive aspects of human milk. Finland went so far as to penalize a non-nursing mother whose child died during the first six months of life.' In Chapter IX, you'll see why that wasn't a bad idea.

The vogue-conscious French almost destroyed their own race in the 18th century when bottle feeding became stylish. A French physician at the time said, "Ladies of quality did not breast feed so they could have more time to

---

* They were, in general, right. See Chapter IX.
** Now that's carrying it a bit far. "Hey Mom, how about breakfast?"

dress, receive and pay visits, attend public shows, and spend the night at their beloved cards."[2]

The history of milk is the history of civilization. Without it there would be no civilization.

REFERENCES

1. La Leche League of New Zealand.
2. Ibid.

Chapter II

UDDER DESTRUCTION
PART I

This is going to be an important chapter. It's the heart of the book. We'll divide it into Part I and Part II.*

A friend of mine in Florida was talking to the wife of a dairyman at a party. My friend, conscious of the myriad of problems associated with pasteurized, homogenized milk, asked her if their dairy would supply her family with raw milk.

The woman blanched white and stiffened. "Certainly not. We would *never touch* the stuff!" The dairyman's wife was offended and embarassed that such a question would be asked in polite company.

When someone that close to milk production has such an emotional and deep-rooted prejudice against fresh milk, the pasteurizers, along with most public health departments and doctors, have indeed convinced the people that heat-treatment of milk, called pasteurization, is as essential as fluoridation of water. But, as with fluoridation, not everybody is convinced. A small band of determined and dedicated dairy farmers and nutritionists continue to work for the return of fresh, untreated "raw" milk.

Initially, the motivation for pasteurization was anything but altruistic. Unscrupulous dairymen knew that if they heated the milk it wouldn't sour, a harmless but often gastronomically undesirable state. Heat treatment enabled them to avoid expensive sanitary procedures and to deliver the milk to unsuspecting consumers apparently "fresh." The milk was anything but fresh; it was

---

*At page 29, take the rest of the day off.

dead. Having killed most of the enzymes and altered the protein and fat through heat, the milk didn't sour-it *rotted* as any dead animal tissue will. However, the dead milk was usually drunk before the rotting process took place, and no one was the wiser. In spite of modern techniques of pasteurization, pasteurized milk is still dead milk which will rot on standing.

People knowledgeable in dairy science at the turn of the century were opposed to heat treatment of milk. They realized that one of nature's almost perfect foods was being altered from a natural food to a processed, unnatural food. During this period, called the "dark era" by pasteurization zealots, conscientious nutritionists and dairy experts strongly opposed pasteurization, realizing that commercial interests were only concerned about shelf life and not nutritious, unadulterated milk.

"Cholera infantum" was a dreaded disease of children in the early 20th century. Five thousand babies died annually from this summer diarrhea. It was found to be caused by milk contaminated by an excessive number of "ordinary dirt bacteria," reported Dr. Park of the New York City Health Department. Just plain dirty milk.

But instead of requiring the dairies to clean up their act, they turned to heat treatment of milk. They eradicated the dreaded "cholera infantum"-but at a terrible price: a steady increase in crib death, infantile allergy, colitis, heart disease, stroke, and sexual impotency, to name a few.

As a *temporary expedient*, while the technologies of sanitation engineering and refrigeration were developing, heat treatment pasteurization was better than nothing. Although the milk was inferior and would cause degenerative diseases later in life, at least it wouldn't kill the children.

But the milk producers are clinging to out-dated methods. In an age of sophisticated sanitation, where even horse liniment and toilet paper are made under remarkably clean conditions, the milk industry leans heavily on heat treatment of milk and milk products to cover up sloppy production methods. This is *sanitation at the wrong end.* The dairymen continue to look backward toward Pasteur and Spallazini rather than forward toward Coit, Mathis, and Steuve. They continue to destroy the food value of milk for economic expediency when, technologically, it is no longer necessary.

Initially, the dairy industry itself also fought the compulsory heating of milk.[1] No one likes to change the system. It costs money. Finally, losing in court, the dairymen caved in and joined the pasteurization movement. Today, locked into the heat pasteurization system, they will fight equally hard to avoid moving forward to fresh, unheated, milk production. The industry continues to "protect" us against disease conditions of one-hundred years ago,* and in the process, they destroy the value of the milk.

In the book *Milk Pasteurization*, Hall and Trout say, "Perhaps no other single innovation has made such an impact on a food industry as the heat treatment of milk. Within the span of one hundred years, the milk industry evolved from almost total obscurity to be the giant of the food industry. The flowering of the milk industry was made possible by the parboiling, or pasteurization as it is now called, of milk."

The parboiling, or heating of milk, had no effect on the incidence of tuberculosis caused by milk.** The incidence of brucellosis, or undulant fever, contrary to popular opinion, was really not affected by the pasteurization process. Brucellosis is not contracted through milk, but

---

* Ask your doctor how many cases of tuberculosis he saw last year.

** You can actually drink milk from a tubercular cow with impunity. The blood-membrane barrier prevents the tubercule bacteria from passing into the milk. It was *tuberculous milkers* who infected the milk by coughing into it.

by association directly with animals. The farmer or other adult milking the cow would often get brucellosis, but his children, *who drank most of the milk,* seldom got the disease.

The so-called pasteurization process is far from new and was done long before Pasteur. In 1782, the Swedish scientist Scheele used heat (pasteurization) treatment to preserve vinegar. In fact, the earliest recorded incidence of the pasteurization process was actually in 1765 by Spallanzini who preserved meat through the heating process.

In 1824, a professor of obstetrics at the University of Pennsylvania, William Dewees, recommended heating milk to the boiling point then cooling for infant feeding. He said, "In hot weather, it is true, the tendency to decomposition is diminished by boiling the milk; but as all the advantages which may result in the process, can be procured without its being absolutely boiled, it should never be had recourse to."

Although Pasteur was given the credit for the parboiling method and it takes its name of pasteurization from him, the record does not show that Louis Pasteur ever pasteurized milk.* Pasteur succeeded in developing a system of heat application to control fermentation and thus the preservation of wine. The wine industry was greatly benefited, as he had discovered the method of preventing wine spoilage. He also succeeded in applying this principle to the preservation of beer. Pasteur does indeed deserve credit, as the basic method applied to milk is the same as that for beer.**

A German, Soxhlat, about twenty years after Pasteur's discovery, applied Pasteur's method to the pasteurization of milk for infant feeding. The process was introduced in the United States in about 1889.

Nathan Straus, a wealthy New York philanthropist, was appalled at the mortality of children being fed raw

---

* I doubt he ever drank it either.
** As with milk, unpasteurized beer is better.

milk. He established milk depots in the city of New York which offered heat-treated milk to children. The death rate from raw milk fell dramatically in New York as a result of Straus' effort Straus spread the gospel around the United States and, in fact, the entire world. He was the single most influential man in making pasteurization a universally used and recognized procedure.

Hall and Trout in their book *Milk Pasteurization* are extremely laudatory of the pasteurization process. They obviously feel that pasteurization is one of the greatest boons ever to come to mankind. The authors list former objections to pasteurization of milk and clearly imply that none of these objections are currently valid. We will list some of these "former objections" and make some comment on them.

- Pasteurization is an excuse for the sale of dirty milk.

- Pasteurization may be used to mask low-quality milk.

- Pasteurization promotes carelessness and discourages the effort to produce clean milk.

- Compulsory pasteurization would diminish the incentive to clean milk production.

- Heat destroys a great number of bacteria in milk and thus conceals the evidence of dirt.

- Pasteurization impairs the flavor of milk.

- Pasteurization diminishes the nutrient value of milk.

- The milk is devitalized.

- Pasteurization diminishes vitamin content.

- Pasteurization destroys Vitamin C.

- Calcium and other minerals are precipitated and made unavailable by pasteurization.

- Milk enzymes are destroyed.

- Infants do not develop well on pasteurized milk.

- Children and infants thrive better on raw milk.

- Pasteurized milk is more likely to lead to decay in teeth.

- Pasteurized milk is more likely to be constipating.

- Pasteurization destroys the creaming ability of milk.

- Pasteurization influences the composition of milk.

- Pasteurization destroys the souring bacteria of milk so that milk instead of souring normally will putrefy if kept long enough.

- Pasteurization kills the bacilli in milk and causes it to decompose when exposed to air. ("bacterial corpse")

- Pasteurization destroys beneficient enzymes, antibodies, and hormones which take the life out of milk.

- Pasteurization may be carelessly done. Therefore, it is not infallible.

- Pasteurized milk may diminish resistance to disease (especially in young babies).

- The death from tuberculosis remains uniformly lower in rural areas where much milk is drunk raw than in cities where all milk is pasteurized.

- Compulsory pasteurization would remove the stimulus to eradicate diseased animals from milking herds.

- Pasteurized milk interferes with the proper development of the teeth and predisposes to dental caries.

- Pasteurization would lead to an increase in infant mortality.

- Pasteurization gives a false sense of security.

There are many others we will not list, but the interesting and important point here is that *all of these "former objections "to pasteurized milk are just as true today as they were when they were listed by Hall and Trout fifteen years ago.* Hall and Trout go on in glowing terms to tell us how three generations have thrived on pasteurized milk and enjoy "radiant health". But they admit, "With so many beliefs unfavorable to the pasteurization of milk, one is astounded that the process was ever introduced. The final acceptance of pasteurization by the consumer is little short of phenomenal."

The state of Massachusetts in 1908, recognizing that pasteurized milk was no longer a vital food, passed a law that required milk subjected to heating to be labeled "heated milk" in one-inch black letters against a white background.

By about 1950 raw certified milk became essentially non-existent in this country, except in three states. The public was thoroughly convinced, through massive advertising over the years, that their original suspicions about pasteurized milk were unfounded, and that the pasteurization process was protecting them from rampant disease conditions. Hall and Trout eulogized, "Pasteurization of milk has attained a near perfection within a half-century. Perhaps the greatest achievement lies in the acclaim of people of many nations for pasteurized household milk."

Although Hall and Trout are extremely laudatory, in fact wildly enthusiastic, about the merits of the pasteurization of milk, they make some interesting comments when comparing the keeping quality of the two types of milk. They say, "The influence . . . on the keeping quality after pasteurization is often exaggerated. The chief organisms responsible for spoilage of pasteurized milk... originate from pasteurization contamination ..."

They go on to quote other authors who concluded that the number of bacteria found in the milk gave absolutely no indication of how well pasteurized milk would keep. As mentioned, the bacteria responsible for spoilage later are not the same ones found in raw milk.

The authors state, apologetically, "The effect of heat for minimum pasteurization intensity has generally little significance, except of course, in the destruction of certain bacteria and enzymes." These "certain bacteria and enzymes" are absolutely vital to the production of nutritious and safe milk. They then go on to admit, because of the complexity of milk fat, that we don't really know how much change takes place due to the pasteurization process. They say, "...milk fat may be involved in many of the unknown effects of heat. Data bearing on the speculative effects of heat on the fat itself are scarcely existent."

The protein casein is also affected by pasteurization. The effects of this on the human body are unknown. They also report that the chief serum proteins of milk, lactalbumin and lactoglobulin, are both adversely affected by high heat treatment of milk. Although the authors admit to the deficiencies of certain vitamins and minerals found in pasteurized milk, they turn to other authorities to reassure us that the changes are negligible. They quote Kay et al, "...the original suggestion that pasteurization seriously diminished the nutritive value of milk has been proved conclusively to be ill-founded."

Enzymes are still little understood as far as their contribution to human nutrition is concerned, but undoubtedly they play an important part. The authors make little of enzymes and report that a large number of enzymes are completely destroyed in the process of pasteurization. They attribute little importance to this and point out that the complete destruction of the enzyme phosphatase is one method of testing to see if the milk has been adequately pasteurized. Phosphatase is essential for the absorption of calcium, *but the complete destruction of phosphatase is the aim of pasteurization!*

The chemistry of calcium in human nutrition is much better understood today than when the phosphatase test was introduced. The "decalcification" of milk which is fed to children may be a major cause of osteoporosis* later in life. We now know that low calcium absorption in healthy women may cause a loss of spinal bone mass as early as age 20.2 Such women may lose 50% or more of their bone mass by the age of 70.**

Other factors which contribute to this literal dissolving of the skeleton are the high phosphates in cola drinks and many food diets, such as the Scarsdale Diet, which is notoriously low in calcium. The high protein diets also accelerate calcium excretion.

When you add other calcium wasting problems such as Vitamin D and C deficiency, alcoholism, antacids, anticoagulants, anticonvulsants, barbiturates, cortisone, diuretics, and smoking, it's no wonder grandma is falling on her face from a fractured hip.***

The enzyme lipase is also totally destroyed by the pasteurization process. Lipase aids in the digestion of fats. Homogenization, the pulverizing of the milk fat,

---

* A thinning of the bones, especially in older women, which leads to fractures, great pain, and premature death.

** That's why fractured hips are a growth industry for the orthopedists.

*** Give her at least a pint of raw milk every day and she will probably never have a fractured hip. She won't waste away either.

causes more lipase to be released into the milk. So, Hall and Trout tell us, "...the complete destruction of lipase (is) imperative; otherwise the milk becomes rancid."

No lipase for fat digestion. No phosphatase for calcium absorption. No galactase for milk sugar digestion. No catalase, diastase, or peroxidase, but the authors conclude, "The healthfulness of people enjoying high per capita consumption of pasteurized milk attest to the maintenance of its nutritive value."

Hall and Trout tell us that, "the Vitamin C content of milk can play an important role in human nutrition." They are referring to pasteurized milk. They claim that a quart of pasteurized milk contains sixteen milligrams of Vitamin C, one-fourth of the official requirement. However, something they did not know at the time was the effect that fluorescent light has on milk. Milk in almost all grocery stores is placed in open bins with fluorescent lighting. This fluorescent lighting has been shown to destroy half of the Vitamin C content of the milk.[3] This loss, along with the pasteurization loss, does not make pasteurized milk a good source of Vitamin C.

In the late 30's, the system of "clarification" was added to the milk processing business. The clarifier is used basically to clean up debris, manure, pus, and other foreign material that is in the milk as a result of sloppy manufacturing methods.

Hall and Trout state, "The centrifugal clarification of milk was early frowned upon by officials who suspected the process would be used to clean up a dirty milk supply." But they say, "Research showed that clarification was necessary to prevent the sedimentation found, even in aseptically produced milk, which was the result of settling out of leucocytes in milk which had been homogenized." The average reader would not know what leucocytes are, so we will tell you: Pus-that's right, just plain pus. With the onset of homogenization, a very undesirable situation had developed. The leucocytes (pus) were noted to settle to the bottom of the bottle and make a greyish oil-like sludge. One cannot sell milk with a pus layer, and, as almost all milk is now homogenized, something had to be done to get this out, so the clarification process was instituted. The sediment removed by the clarification process is called in the milk trade, slime-and that is exactly what it is.*

One reason for the accumulation of pus and other slime elements in the milk is the current method of delivering milk to the processing centers. The milk may be picked up at the farm daily, but it goes into a holding tank and is only bottled three times a week. It may be *four or five days old* when finally bottled.** If it wasn't "clarified" and pasteurized at the processing center, it would be a lethal brew on delivery to the supermarket.

Raw certified milk could be kept four to five days with absolutely no damage to the public because it is clean when milked. But it is delivered in less than twenty-four hours from milking to the consumer.

In one investigation detailing the "heat treatment" of milk, it was revealed that not just one simple heating takes place. Milk is heated over again with each process. In clarification, the milk may be heated to 135° Fahrenheit. In the filtering process, the milk is heated again to about 100° Fahrenheit. In the bactofugation process (method of removing bacteria), the milk is again heated to 170° Fahrenheit. With deaeration a vacuum treatment is used in which the milk is treated in two vacuum chambers, the first at 175° Fahrenheit, the second at 100°-152° Fahrenheit.*** These heats may vary according to the system used, but the milk is heated over and over again. It is hard to imagine this milk resembling the original product after all of this steam-cleaning.

---

* A process called vacuration removes undesirable odors from dirty milk. That's why those in the business call the vacurator a "fart snatcher."

** The date on the carton is calculated from the *time of bottling*, not the time of milking.

*** Bulk storage of milk has led to off-flavor (tainting). Food Engineering Magazine has the answer: "Blanching", which means heating the milk again!

In the old days, doctors and scientists had a clear understanding of the milk problem. It's peculiar how old truths have to be rediscovered. In 1926, an ordinance was proposed in Missouri that would have prohibited the sale of raw milk. The judge in the case said:*

> "A great volume of evidence was offered regarding the relative qualities of raw milk and pasteurized milk. A large number of practicing physicians, chemists, bacteriologists, and users of milk were sworn. The evidence conclusively shows that pasteurization altered the character of the milk, and the testimony of far the greater number of physicians and bacteriologists who testified was that pasteurization impairs its quality; that it destroys some of the vitamins in the milk and impairs others; that it destroys the lactic acid which causes milk to sour; that souring is a process of self-preservation; and lactic acid is an important element in counteracting pernicious bacteria; that pasteurization disintegrates the salts, such as calcium, iron, and phosphates, causes them to lose their organic quality and makes them more difficult, if not impossible, to assimilate; that pasteurization caused constipation and indigestion particularly among babies and children; that it breaks down the enzymes, though other physicians said there was sufficient of that element in the digestive organisms of persons who drink milk. It was shown that doctors generally require raw milk for ailing babies and children; that children who could not flourish on pasteurized milk usually improved in health and flourished on raw milk. There was other evidence to show that one reason for the satisfactory healthfulness of raw milk is that it increases the vitality and resistance of a child because it is easier to assimilate; that the destruction of pathogenic germs by pasteurization was more than counterbalanced by the superior quality of raw milk.
>
> In addition to the professional evidence offered, the relators offered the testimony of a number of mothers and other raisers of children, and they uniformly testified that children who were not healthful when fed on

---

*Judges can be boring, but this one isn't. Read on.

pasteurized milk were healthful when fed raw milk. The respondents made no attempt to counteract that testimony, but countenance it was unimportant coming from non-professional source. But it was the opinion of several Physicians that actual experience' particularly clinical experience, was more valuable than laboratory tests in determining the effects of milk upon the system. "*

The court decided that the ordinance prohibiting the sale of raw milk was in conflict with the law and should be invalidated.

A letter written to the Journal of the American Veterinarian Medical Association by Dr. Edward T. Henry, D.V.M., contained the usual arguments that pasteurized homogenized milk is as nutritious as fresh milk. Dr. Henry says, ". . . Let me lay to rest the myth that pasteurization lowers the nutrition of milk. True, several enzymes and maybe a vitamin or two are destroyed, but one should not be relying totally on milk for those constituents. *Pasteurization has very little, if any, effect on the nutritional value of dairy products.*"

Dr. Henry raises the spector in his letter of the host of diseases one may contract if one drinks raw certified milk. He states, ". . . the consuming public can be guaranteed that the milk they are purchasing, if pasteurized, is free of disease-causing microorganisms, such as brucellosis, tuberculosis, paratyphoid fever, typhoid fever, salmonellosis, shigellosis, Q fever, just to name a few."

Some of these diseases, such as Q fever and brucellosis, never did come from contaminated milk.**

"When consuming raw milk", he continued, "who can be absolutely sure it is free of the foregoing microorganisms? These are diseases that can kill and some peo-

---

* Case number and judge's name are unknown.
** Q fever is an airborne virus contracted through the respiratory system.

ple want to allow use of raw milk-all in the name of freedom of choice. Even with all the testing of both cows and milk, people who drink raw milk are exposing themselves to potential life-threatening diseases."

This technique of pointing with horror at non-existent problems has undoubtedly discouraged many people from drinking unprocessed milk. The many years of consumption of raw certified milk by tens of thousands proves beyond a doubt, that the terrible spector raised by Dr. Henry simply does not exist.

But the Council on Public Health and Regulatory Veterinary Medicine continued the myth by passing a resolution in 1979 condemning the use of raw milk on the basis that it was unsafe, "Only pasteurized milk and milk products should be sold for human consumption." This resolution indicates the rampant ignorance and prejudice existing concerning the modern production of unprocessed milk. This ignorance and prejudice is not only present in the veterinary field, but is almost universally found in the field of human medicine.

Back in the days of our Pilgrim fathers tomatoes were considered poisonous. One iconoclastic gentleman ate a tomato in public to disprove the superstition. Everyone thought he was committing suicide. He survived the experiment, but it didn't change anybody's mind.*

The tomato story has it's modern counterpart. Paul Virgin of the Alta-Dena Dairy drinks raw milk on television to prove that raw milk contains no evil spirits. In contrast, homogenized, pasteurized milk is an unhealthy product as shown by many tests. The avoidance of nutritious, safe, raw, certified milk today because of previous disease conditions that no longer exist is as absurd as it would be not to eat tomatoes in the 20th century because they were considered to be poisonous in the 17th century.

---

* If he had been a woman, they would have burned him at the stake for witchcraft.

It is surprising that pasteurization caught on, as most knowledgeable milk scientists at the time did all they could to ferret out the pasteurizers who operated illegally and undercover. But the milk lobby eventually won and made the process respectable. In 1947 Michigan passed a compulsory pasteurization law and the rest of the nation rapidly capitulated. Junk milk, by 1960, was compulsory in almost every state.

The dairy industry is committing suicide. Milk consumption is decreasing relative to the growth of the population.* The reasons are:

1) The false propaganda about cholesterol and fat causing hardening of the arteries (heart attacks, strokes) promulgated by the news media with the blessing of organized medicine.

2) Many people simply don't like the taste of heatprocessed milk. One reason pasteurized milk doesn't taste like milk back on the farm is because of the practice of "holding over" milk. The milk is placed in large "raw milk silos" until ready for processing. It may stay there for days. This favors the growth of bacteria called psychrotrophics.[4] These bacteria grow quite nicely at the refrigeration temperatures of the silos used for storage. The psychrotrophics produce enzymes that are extremely heat-resistant and easily survive the pasteurization process. That's why your pasteurized milk may taste bitter, unclean, oily, chalky, metallic or medicinal.**

3) The serious allergies that heat-processed milk has caused among children and adults alike. Pasteurized milk allergy, caused by altering the milk proteins through heating, has caused a major health problem in the United States.

---

* From 1970 to 1980 whole milk consumption decreased 33%.
** Yuck. No wonder people have stopped drinking milk.

4) The growing realization among consumers that processed food, including pasteurized homogenized milk, is a health hazard.

In this modern world, yesterday's crime, such as abortion, becomes today's essential service. Pasteurization was a crime at the turn of the century and the pasteurizer had to lurk in the dark to kill milk. Although all of the sophisticated biochemical knowledge that we have today was not available to them, milk experts knew that heating milk, as in the pasteurization process, was changing a live food into a dead food and was simply a cop-out for the dairy farmer. It's much cheaper to make dirty milk and then kill most of the bacteria by heating than to maintain a clean dairy with clean cows and clean milk.

Figure 1 on the following page would indicate that since pasteurization of milk, infant mortality has steadily declined. In 1908 there were seventy-five infant deaths per thousand. In 1970 there were only ten. But, if this graph is expanded, as in Figure 2, it is immediately obvious that pasteurization probably had little to do with the drop in infant mortality. There had been a steady decline in infant mortality since the middle 1700's.

The greatest contribution to eradication of infectious diseases was the automobile. The automobile has given us a lot of pollution but it replaced a far worse pollution-the horse.

It's hard for modern man to imagine how filthy the big cities were when everything in the city moved by horse. People, rich and poor, virtually waded through a sea of horse manure. With the manure came flies-billions of them. With the flies came infectious diseases, the major cause of death until the mid twentieth century. Only the hardy survived, which is probably the main reason man eventually triumphed over infections. But the elimination of the horse from areas of high population density was a major factor. It is also interesting to note, return-

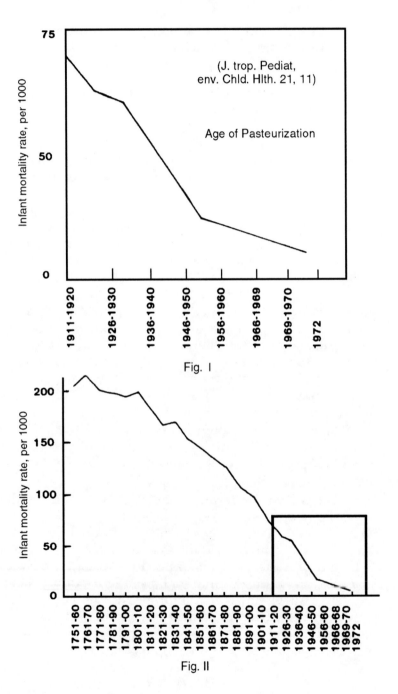

Fig. I

Fig. II

ing to Figure 2, that the boxed-in area also represents the age of immunization and antibiotic therapy. The period of greatest usage of antibiotics has been from 1950 to the present. As the graph illustrates, the rate of decline in infant mortality has been actually less since the advent of the miracle drugs.

Dr. J.M. Prucha, professor emeritus in dairy bacteriology, University of Illinois, said forty years ago, *"There was much opposition to pasteurization of milk and at best, it was looked upon as a temporary expedient to obtain a safe milk supply until the time when the dairy industry would learn to produce clean and safe milk."*[5] (Emphasis added.)

The propaganda that pasteurized milk is safer than fresh raw certified milk can be easily put to rest. In 1945 there were four hundred fifty cases of infectious disease caused by raw milk. There were one thousand four hundred ninety two cases caused by pasteurized milk.[6] Knowing that statistics don't lie and statisticians do,-let's look at the figures from a different angle. There was one case of disease for every twelve million four hundred thousand quarts of pasteurized milk consumed and one case of disease for every eighteen million nine hundred thousand quarts of raw milk consumed.' In other words, you could drink six million five hundred thousand more quarts of raw milk than pasteurized without getting sick!

In 1945 there was an epidemic of food poisoning in Phoenix, Arizona.[8] The official report reads, "Pasteurization charts... show milk was properly pasteurized and leads to the assumption that toxin was produced in milk while it was stored without refrigeration and *was not completely destroyed by pasteurization"*-three hundred very sick people from pasteurized milk.

Great Bend, Kansas, same year, had four hundred sixtyeight cases of gastroenteritis from pasteurized milk. This was traced to "unsanitary conditions in dairies, unsterilized bottles, improper pasteurization." Nine died.

June, 1982. Over one hundred seventy-two people in a three state area in the Southeast were stricken with an intestinal infection. Over one hundred required hospitalization. The infection, which caused severe diarrhea, fever, nausea, abdominal pain, and headache, was caused by pasteurized milk.[9]

Does this happen today? Of course it does, but doctors and parents are unlikely to blame milk because, after all, it is *pasteurized*. They will blame Junior's gastroenteritis and diarrhea on everything but contaminated, pasteurized milk.*

The toxin from bacteria largely responsible for diarrhea, the enterotoxin, is *largely unaffected* by pasteurization.[10] If raw milk is contaminated to a significant degree you can tell it instantly from the smell and taste. But pasteurized milk may be seriously contaminated with no tell-tale odor at all.

Consumer Reports of January, 1974, revealed how shoddy milk production is in the United States. Out of one hundred twenty-five samples of milk and milk products, forty-four percent proved to be in violation of state regulations. Consumer Reports concluded, "The quality of a number of the dairy products in this study was little short of deplorable." Consumer's Union, reporting in June, 1982, stated that fecal bacteria, called coliforms, were found in many samples tested. Some had counts as high as 2200 organisms per cubic centimeter. Raw certified milk must contain no more than 10 coliforms per cubic centimeter.**

As we stated earlier and confirmed by Consumer Reports, the "former objections" to pasteurized milk are just as valid today:

   a) Pasteurization is an excuse for the sale of dirty
      milk.

----

* The next time you have diarrhea, test your pasteurized milk. See Appendix II for the method.

** The same standard is supposed to apply to pasteurized milk, but who's checking?

b) Pasteurization may be used to mask low quality milk.

c) Pasteurization promotes carelessness and discourages the effort to produce clean milk.

Professor Fosgate, of the Dairy Science Department of the University of Georgia, spoke out on pasteurization, "Pasteurization has been preached as a one-hundred percent safeguard for milk. This simply is not true. *If milk gets contaminated today, the chances are that it will be after pasteurization. Pasteurized milk and raw milk are equally susceptible to contamination by pathogenic bacteria...*" (Emphasis added.)

Fosgate is probably too conservative. Raw milk contains enzymes and antibodies, destroyed by pasteurization, that make it less susceptible to bacterial contamination. But, Dr. Fosgate stands up for Rosebud and the rest of America's milk-producing ruminants, "The dairy cow has been sadly maligned by the dairy and food industry in general. She has been pictured as a veritable 'Typhoid Mary' for all of the ills of man, including the common cold, when actually, the reverse is true." The full import of this statement will be brought out in the chapter on milk as a therapeutic agent in disease.

Other than the greater infectious potential of pasteurized milk, are there other disadvantages to processed milk? Enough to fill a few chapters. But before we go on to other disadvantages of pasteurized milk, let's look at an example of the amazing protective qualities of raw milk, even when it's dirty.

Jack Mathis, President of Atlanta's Mathis Dairy, was invited to inspect the dairy at the Atlanta City Prison Farm and make suggestions for modernization. He found the entire operation to be indescribably filthy. "It looked more like an outhouse than a milking parlor," was his first observation. The pathetic cows were in obvious pain, being milked by machines entirely unattended.

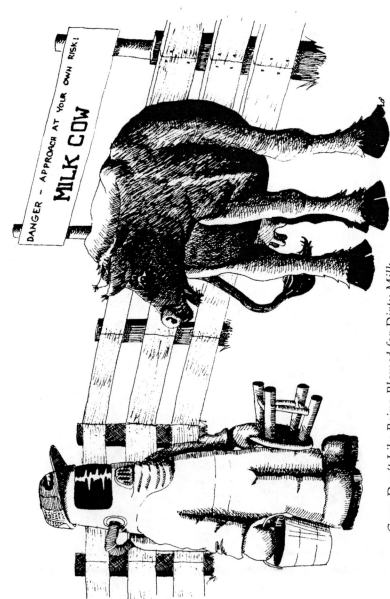

Cows Don't Like Being Blamed for Dirty Milk.

Manure on the cow's hindquarters was running over the teats, the milking apparatus, and into the milk. From the milking machine, the milk ran into an open ten-gallon can by hose. "You couldn't see the top of the can for the flies," Mathis said. "It was like a bee hive with flies walking in and out of the can."

Jack Mathis assumed that the milk was for the prison farm pigs, but it wasn't. It went directly to a cooler in the prison dining hall, complete with cow and fly manure and fly carcases. It was simply strained through the cooler and then drunk by the prisoners.

No one had gotten sick from the milk in ten years. What a case for raw milk!

REFERENCES

1. Bartlett, R.W., The Milk Industry, pp. 254, Ronald Press Company, New York City, New York, 1946.
2. Medical Month, January 1964, pp. 43.
3. "Public Health Report," U.S. Public Health Service, 1945.
4. Dairy Record, February, 1982.
5. Milk Facts, Milk Industry Foundation, New York City, 1946-47.
6. Ibid.
7. Fosgate letter.
8. Darlington, pp. 21 and 19.
9. The Atlanta Journal, Atlanta, Georgia, September 24, 1982.
10. AAMMC Annual Conference, Kansas City, Missouri, May 1976.

Chapter III

UDDER DESTRUCTION
PART II

One Friday morning when I was in medical school, a group of eight farm workers who had been spraying vegetables were brought to the emergency department of the university hospital. They were all dead but one. The one survivor lived only because he had been thrown in the truck upside down. The others died of pulmonary edema -drowning from fluid in their lungs. The one lucky worker drained his lungs spontaneously because of being upsidedown and so he survived.

The chemical causing this disaster is known as an organo-phosphate. You wouldn't want that in your milk, would you? Many dairies are now feeding an organo-phosphate to their cattle. This chemical, known as lincophos, ends up in the manure and poisons the larvae of flies. Isn't that clever? Why maintain a clean barn when you can just dose your cows with organo-phosphate and let the chemically contaminated manure poison the maggots? What does this dosing with chemicals do to the cow and the cow's milk? The FDA says it does nothing. They've told us that before.*

The average commercial dairy farmer is interested primarily in production figures rather than quality. Those farmers who are sincerely concerned about the drastic decline in the quality of milk can do little about it until the public demands a better product. The farmer sells to

---

*Remember DES, swine flue vaccine, and Oraflex?

a vast consortium and has no control over the final product that may look the same as the milk from his cow, but bio-chemically, enzymatically, and nutritionally is about as close to real milk as "non-dairy creamer" is to real cream.

The farmer wants pituitary-giant freaks that produce their body weight in milk every ten days. But the milk from these milk-producing superstars may contain excessive amounts of pituitary hormones.

The pituitary excretion affecting growth is called the "growth hormone." This hormone may account for the fact that each succeeding generation of Americans for the past fifty years has been taller than their parents. This excess height, although associated with handsomeness and health in our culture, may actually be a sign of abnormal pituitary function due to excess pituitary growth hormone from milk. Bigger is not necessarily healthier.

The independent dairy farmer producing raw, certified milk is interested in quality as well as quantity. He knows that these abnormal milk producers are prone to be unhealthy and subject to infection requiring the frequent use of antibiotics. As he doesn't cover mistakes and unsanitary production methods by heat-treating the milk, he is more likely to own normal, healthy cows producing less milk but without excess pituitary and other hormones.

The pituitary also stimulates the production of sex hormones. Could this be contributing to the vast array of sexual problems we see today? Sexual dysfunction has become so common that the medical profession now has a separate journal to deal with it.

There is some connection, not yet entirely understood, between certain cancers and hormones. Pasteurized milk is apparently adding to the problem as there is a relationship between certain types of cancer and the consumption of pasteurized milk.

The pituitary hormone, TSH, stimulates the thyroid gland. If minute amounts of this pituitary hormone were to be absorbed daily from unbalanced pasteurized milk, depression of the thyroid gland could eventually result. Low thyroid function has become extremely common in this country. Some experts estimate that fifty percent of the people over fifty years of age have some degree of low functioning thyroid. Could milk from pituitary-giant cows be contributing to the problem?

Another hormone, from the pituitary, ADH, causes water retention. Two other hormones work directly on the ovaries and the testicles and may also contribute to several dysfunctions. ACTH, a powerful adrenal stimulator, can cause everything from diabetes and hypertension to Addison's Disease (adrenal exhaustion), and acne.

Through the process of chromotography, we now know that synthetic vitamins are not the same as natural ones. The pasteurizers love to point out the vitamin content of their heat-treated milk, using this as an argument for equivalent nutrient value between natural, raw, certified milk and heated, pasteurized milk. But Vitamin C, for instance, is higher in concentration in fresh raw milk than in heat-treated, pasteurized milk - 33% more. The pasteurization fanatics quickly point out that "both are inadequate in Vitamin C, and neither raw or pasteurized milk should be depended upon as a Vitamin C source." If this is true, why do babies fed pasteurized milk develop a scurvy-like syndrome and raw milk-fed babies do not?

Pottenger proved there is a yet undiscovered deficiency disease, similar to Vitamin C deficiency (scurvy), that can be cured by giving an endocrine product *that contains no Vitamin C*.[2] Raw milk has this unknown nutrient and pasteurized milk does not. Stefansson, a famous arctic explorer, demonstrated that a supposedly adequate intake of Vitamin C in the form of tomato juice did not prevent scurvy in an arctic sea captain.[3] Whereas just a few days on raw meat cured him completely. As shown by Pottenger, raw milk, if it had been available, would have accomplished the same thing.

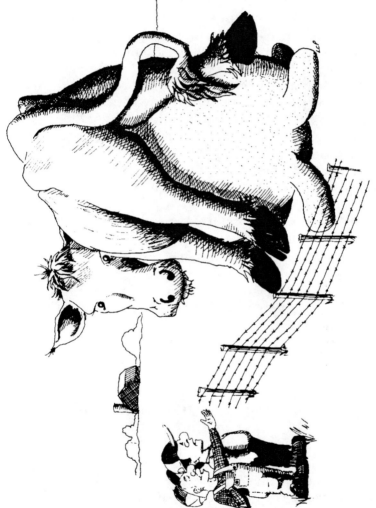

Pituitary Giant Freaks Produce More Milk. But What About the Quality?

It was pointed out in 1942 that "...the cows of the country *produce as much Vitamin C as does the entire citrus crop,* but most of it is lost as the result of pasteurization."[4]

Today the losses in commercial pasteurized milk are even greater. Jack Jansen, Ph.D., Clemson University Department of Dairy Science, studied the vitamin losses in milk stored in translucent plastic jugs and exposed to continuous fluorescent lighting.[5] This merchandising practice is standard today in most supermarkets. Jansen found that at least half of the Vitamin C content of the milk was destroyed after twenty-four hours of the light exposure. An interesting additional finding of the Jansen study was that the fluorescent lighting caused a "light-induced oxidized flavor." Taste tests of Clemson students revealed that they preferred the oxidized taste and accepted it as the real taste of milk!

The work of Friedberger is intensely interesting in this regard.[6] Friedberger found that heat treatment actually caused deficiencies not caused by vitamin destruction. The vitamins were certainly destroyed, but animals on the heat-processed product *with vitamins added* still reacted adversely just like those not receiving any additional vitamins at all.

What Pasteurized, Homogenized Milk Can Do To You

In Chapter XI we report on how raw milk and immunized raw milk often can give great benefit to the sufferer of rheumatoid arthritis and other diseases. You also need to know what the wrong kind of milk can do to you.

It's chilling to read the findings from the Korean War[7] which vividly illustrate the degeneration of American youth. Of the young men killed there, autopsy examination revealed that 12% had a 50% blockage of the arteries of the heart. Five percent of them had blockage of

90%. Remember, these were young men in their teens and twenties. Do you think we have a problem? We're in the third generation of degeneration, like Doctor Pottenger's experimental cats. (See Chapter XI).

Skim or low-fat milk may cause degenerative arthritis, also called hypertrophic or calcific arthritis. Calcification of other tissues such as the pineal gland, arteries, and kidneys may also be caused by drinking fractionated (skim, non-fat) milk.

There is a little gland right dead center in the skull called the pineal gland. We were taught in medical school that the pineal gland was unimportant as it had no function; one of those little mistakes of evolution. Ancient philosophers thought the pineal was the site of the soul.*

This little gland is often calcified, even in young people but, as it had no function, nobody cared whether it was calcified or not. We now know that the pineal gland is extremely important in light physiology and hormonal regulation, especially in women.

Calcification of the arteries (arteriosclerosis), the joints (degenerative arthritis), and this important gland may be due to the excessive intake of fractionated milk, i.e., skim or low-fat milk. On the advice of physicians, millions of people have switched to low-fat milk under the mistaken belief that avoiding the milk fat will enable them to avoid hardening of the arteries. Drinking fractionated milk may cause exactly the opposite effect!

Many other millions are drinking low-fat milk to avoid weight gain. This practice, combining a low carbohydrate diet and skim milk, is used by most of the popular weight reduction clinics around the country.**

---

* Organized religion has taken a stand against this theory, and recent scientific investigation has revealed some other uses for the pineal gland.

** Do you know how a farmer fattens his hogs? He feeds them skim milk.

The Wulzen Calcium Dystrophy Syndrome may sound a long way away from your local fat farm, but it is closer than you think. Wulzen did her classic experiments in the 30's. Her results have tremendous clinical significance in human nutrition, but, like Crewe's work with milk therapy, they have been largely ignored.[8]

Wulzen reported that guinea pigs fed fresh raw milk thrived and at autopsy showed no abnormalities of any kind. The test animals fed pasteurized milk did not grow well and consistently developed a highly characteristic syndrome, the first sign of which was wrist stiffness, a form of arthritis. But far worse was the effects from pasteurized, skim milk. These animals not only did not do well,-they became weak and emaciated and then died. First they developed the characteristic wrist stiffness and then muscular dystrophy. Autopsy revealed severe hardening of the arteries and calcification of other soft tissues. In humans this syndrome is probably manifested by calcification of the joints, which we know as degenerative arthritis, hardening of the arteries, cataract, and calcification of that important gland, the pineal.

Wulzen postulated that there was an "anti-stiffness factor" in the cream portion of the milk. She later proved that this factor is a steroid, a cortisone-like chemical. If the animals were fed raw cream or a carbohydrate, the wrist stiffness would be reversed. Lack of carbohydrate will increase the symptoms. This may be highly significant in our diet-conscious and forever-reducing population.

The "anti-stiffness factor" is probably not the only substance in the cream that remains undiscovered. When animals are placed on skim milk with the vitamins lost from the cream replaced, the animals develop very poorly. But when four percent butter fat is fed to similar animals, they develop normally. The vegetable oils now being pushed on the American people by organized medicine and self-styled nutrition experts will not work as a substitute for cream.

Skim milk-fed animals develop testicular atrophy with complete sterility. Male sterility is a major concern in our country today, and the skim milk fad may be a major contributing factor.

The test animals also developed severe calcification of most large blood vessels, anemia, and high blood pressure. Another characteristic of the syndrome that may be of significance in human medicine is the development of calcium deposits around the bone openings in the spine that provide for the exit of nerves. Sciatica and other nerve compression syndromes may be caused by this nutritional deficiency. Also, a decrease in hearing, leading to complete deafness was consistently found.

How much of Wulzen's findings in guinea pigs apply to man is not known. But the implications are too ominous to ignore. People who drink skim or low-fat milk, and millions have switched, are usually calorie and weight-conscious. So the skim milk they drink plus a low-carbohydrate diet may be contributing to the extensive calcific degeneration we now see in so many patients.

Critics say that just because we see this calcification in guinea pigs doesn't mean it happens to people. But who has offered any well-documented, experimental proof of any other cause for the extensive calcific disease that we see today? Other dietary factors may contribute to this calcification, such as excess sugar consumption, heated protein foods such as meat, chlorinated and fluoridated water, magnesium deficiency, thyroid deficiency secondary to iodine deficiency, xanthine oxidase, smoking, cadmium poisoning, and so on. But the Wulzen experiments were conclusive and *repeatable*.

A Dutch chemist, Willem J. VanWagtendork at Oregon State College, confirmed the Wulzen findings. He found that guinea pigs with calcification of the tissues could be relieved with raw cream. The active factor is killed by pasteurization. Professor Hugo Kruger of Oregon State University again confirmed Wulzen's experiments. He proved that there is a definite connection between pasteurized milk and stiff joints which eventually leads, in experimental animals, to muscular dystrophy.

With all this evidence indicating that pasteurized milk, especially skim, will turn you into stone, wouldn't you think that nutritional leaders would be promoting raw milk?

Granted, most of the experiments have been done with experimental animals, but as the great French physiologist, Rene Dubos said, "From the point of view of scientific philosophy, the largest achievement of modern biochemistry has been the demonstration *of the fundamental unity* of the chemical processes associated with life." In other words, if it happens in guinea pigs, it probably will happen to you.

R.D. Briggs of the Pathology Department of Washington University School of Medicine, reading that the British had reported a higher incidence of heart attacks among persons with chronic peptic ulcers, 9 hypothesized that this increased incidence may be due to the treatment, specifically, the ingestion of large quantities of milk.[10]

Briggs and his associates undertook a statistical study of ten medical centers in the United States and five in Great Britain. They compared the incidence of heart attacks in ulcer patients taking a Sippy (pasteurized, homogenized milk and cream) diet with those not using milk. Their results were startling and unequivocal. In the United States, patients taking the Sippy diet had a threefold higher incidence of heart attacks. In England the heavy pasteurized, homogenized milk drinkers had a sixfold increase in heart attacks as compared to the non-milk users.

In their discussion, Briggs, et al comment, "Even if the increased intake of milk is responsible for the higher incidence of myocardial infarction in ulcer patients, the identity of the specific constituent of milk that is important in this respect has not yet been established."

That was 1960. We now know from the work of Pottenger, Wulzen, McCulley, Oster, and others what the "specific constituents" are: heated protein and xanthine oxidase. Natural milk, raw milk, contains no heated protein and no biologically available xanthine oxidase.

The Sudden Infant Death Syndrome (SID), also called "crib death," has baffled scientists for years. An apparently healthy baby dies in its sleep, without crying, without struggling. These infants are six months of age or younger with the highest incidence at about three months. Almost every conceivable cause, from Vitamin C deficiency (probable), to suffocation from bedding (unlikely), has been hypothesized as the cause of this tragic form of death in apparently healthly infants.

Barrett, in 1954, suggested that inhalation of food while sleeping may be the cause. This could never be demonstrated at autopsy. But Barrett and his co-workers at the University of Cambridge then went a little deeper into the inhaled food theory.

It had already been proven that most infants fed on cow milk have evidence, in their blood, that they are potentially allergic to cow milk protein. Infants often regurgitate various amounts of milk while asleep. If a child has built up a strong sensitivity to cow milk, they reasoned, then why couldn't he experience a massive allergic reaction, analphylactic shock, to a small amount of milk inhaled into the lungs?

Using guinea pigs, they set out to test this theory. Guinea pigs were sensitized to milk. Then the animals were subjected to cow milk dripped into the throat and down the windpipe. The effect, although dramatic and devastating, was not like the quiet "slipping away" of the child who dies in the night from SID without a whimper. The animals convulsed violently and then died, hardly a "slipping away."

Back to the drawing board. Why was the reaction different? The blood antibodies were present in the animals. The reaction should have been the same as in humans. Something was missing.

"Wait!" a bright researcher said, "the babies die in their *sleep*. No one has ever *seen* a baby die of the Sudden Infant Death Syndrome. They don't die in their mother's arms. They always die when no one is around, while sleeping."

Okay, let's anesthetize the animals, they reasoned. This will simulate the sleep condition of infants who die of the "crib death."

The results were startling and unequivocal, *"Very soon after introducing the milk into the larynx of an anesthetized guinea pig, the animal stopped breathing* **without any sign of struggle.** Death was preceded by a short period of more rapid breathing... until, with a final nose-twitching, the animal died."

Their conclusion, "It has thus been demonstrated that sensitized animals, when unconscious, *can be killed quickly, silently, and without trace of struggle* by the inhalation of whole milk..." (Emphasis added.)*

In classic British understatement they added, "...the fact that babies do become sensitized to cow milk protein, and that inhalation of this material could conceivably be the cause of crib death in a young infant, should be another inducement to breast-feed young babies where practicable."

As breast-fed babies rarely die of Sudden Infant Death Syndrome, we would suggest that babies should be breast-fed whether "practicable" or not. Suggestions:

1) Insist that your baby be put immediately to breast, the mother's breast, after birth.

2) *Get the advice of an experienced midwife or mother* concerning breast feeding or contact LaLeche League. The average doctor knows little or nothing about

---

* On vitamin C deficiency as a cause of SID, see "Every Second Child," Kalokerinos, Keats Publishing, New Canaan, Conn.

breast feeding and may give you bad advice (if he gives you any at all).

3) *Beware of baby formula propaganda.* Don't be fooled by the numbers game they play in comparing the constituents in mother's milk and formula.

4) *Gain adequate weight for breast feeding* during pregnancy. A breast-feeding mother can lose significant amounts of calcium and other nutrients if she doesn't lay up plenty of fat prior to delivery.

We'll tell you more about breast milk in Chapter IX.

Although pasteurized milk is promoted by its manufacturers as being essential for good teeth, a number of investigations would indicate otherwise. The studies of Steinman in California are particularly relevant."

Steinman studied rats. The decay process in rats' teeth is biologically identical to that in human teeth. He divided his rats into several groups. The control group received a standard nutritious rat chow made by the Purina Company. These rats, Steinman discovered, would average less than one cavity for their entire lifetime. The second group received a very heavy refined sugar diet. Although they grew faster than the Purina rats, they averaged 5.6 cavities per rat.

Now the shocker. The third group was fed "homogenized grade A pasteurized milk" and *they had almost twice as many cavities as the sugar-fed group* — 9.4 cavities per animal.*

If processed milk does this to your teeth, what does it do to your other high-calcium organ-your bones? How does it affect calcium metabolism in the soft tissues of the body such as the blood vessels?

---

* You think that's bad? Add chocolate to Junior's pasteurized homogenized Grade A milk and the cavity rate quadruples overthat of the sugar diet.

Remember that your teeth are the window to your body's physical condition. They reflect your general state of health. If your teeth are deteriorating, *you* are deteriorating. Hardening of the arteries and decaying teeth are part of the same degenerative process. The one you can see, cavities, comes early in life. The other, atherosclerosis- heart attack, is not seen and comes later. They are a *continuum* - part of the same degenerative process leading to disease and death.

Dr. Weston Price in his masterpiece, *Nutrition and Human Degeneration* proved fifty years ago what Steinman showed in 1963: Processed food leads to disease and premature death.[12]

Milk contains a lot of sugar. But milk sugar, called lactose, doesn't have the same poisonous side effects as regular sugar, sucrose. It is more slowly absorbed into the blood stream, and so it doesn't jolt the pancreas into oversecretion of insulin which leads to hypoglycemia and, eventually, diabetes.

But, after pasteurization, you have a different story. Heating the milk turns the lactose into beta-lactose which is far more soluble and therefore more rapidly absorbed into the blood stream. The sudden rise in blood sugar is followed by a fall leading to low blood sugar, hypoglycemia, which induces hunger. If more milk is drunk to satisfy the hunger, then the cycle is repeated: hyperglycemia - hypoglycemia-hunger-more milk, etc. The end result is obesity. Obesity has become one of the most common diseases of childhood. Pasteurized milk makes you fat; raw milk does not.*

The switch to pasteurized, heat-treated milk gave a great impetus to the milk industry at the turn of the century. People were confident that milk was nutritious and safe. But with the increase in consumption of pasteurized milk came a dramatic and steady increase in arthritis,

---

*Unless you really pig out.

heart disease, crib death, and stroke. Now people again have become suspicious of processed pasteurized milk.

The milk industry is indeed committing suicide. The use of fluid milk is on the decline both in total quantity and per capita usage.[13] The abandonment of raw milk is a national tragedy. Fresh, unadulterated milk is largely unavailable except in two states. The producers, having ruined milk through processing, leave the people with two choices: (1) Drink milk that many experts say will ruin their health; (2) Abstain from drinking milk.

The end result is clear: The eventual disappearance of a nutritious food resource-natural milk. A great physician predicted twenty years ago:

"Unless the dairy industry is to awaken ...it will give sway to the chemist and engineer and forget that, so far, only God has made life. Like dogs and horses, the dairy cow will become the pet of the curious, to be preserved in zoos like the Texas Longhorn."

REFERENCES

1. Darlington, pp. 21, 19.

2. AAMMC Annual Conf., Kansas City, Missouri, May 1976.

3. Harper's Magazine, November/December, 1925 & January 1936.

4. Proc. Nat. Nut Conf. for Defence, May 14, Federal Sea Agency, pp. 176; U.S. Government Pat. Off., 1942.

5. Family Practice News, September 1, 1981.

6. Certified Milk Magazine, October 1927 as reported by Victor E. Levine, Prof. of Biological Chemistry Nutrition, Creighton University School of Medicine.

7. Enos, et al, JAMA, 158;912, 1955.

8. Amer. J. Physical, 133-500, 1941; Physiol. Zool., 8:457, 1935.

9. Morris, Brit. M.J., 2:1485, 1958.

10. Circulation, Vol. XXI, pp. 438, April 1960.

11. So. Cal. State Dent. Assoc. J., Vol. XXXI, Nr. 9, September 1963.

12. Price-Pottenger Foundation, La Mesa, California.

13. Pottenger, Clinical Physiology, Volume III, Nr. 3, 1961.

Chapter IV
UDDER PROPAGANDA

Picture a milk bottle with a skull and crossbones on it and the title, "Raw Milk Can Kill You." That's pretty heavy stuff for Coronet Magazine. But that's what they hit the American people with in May, 1945.

"Crossroads, U.S.A., is in one of those states in the Midwest area called the breadbasket and milk bowl of America. Crossroads lies about twenty-five miles from the big city on a good paved highway... What happened to Crossroads might happen to your town ... might happen almost anywhere in America." Coronet's expert, Dr. Harold Harris, then went on to describe in livid detail the epidemic of undulant fever in Crossroads that infected twenty-five percent of the population and killed one in four. Case histories were then given to show how subtle and debilitating the disease could be.

Investigation revealed that twenty-five percent of the population of Crossroads did not get undulant fever, and one out of four infected did *not* die *because the town of "Crossroads "does not even exist!* The entire article, because of the harm it did to the raw milk industry, and indirectly to the health of the American people, was more irresponsible than yelling "fire" in a crowded theatre.

"A curious incident in New York City," Harris tells his wide-eyed readers, "concerned a physician who fell ill of brucellosis.', Wham-within a few days he was dead. The source of his lethal infection of undulant fever, or brucellosis, was cheese "dripping with germs," Harris reported.

The incident was indeed "curious" in that: 1) Undulant fever doesn't cause death in a few days, 2) Cheese does not transmit undulant fever, and 3) Investigation through the New York City Health Department revealed that there was no such case ever reported! Harris puts forth so many outlandish claims and preposterous misstatements that one wonders if he bothered to do any research at all and, if he did, if he didn't just decide to ignore the facts and write a sensational article that would sell to a major magazine, and scare the pants off people drinking raw milk. Harris either made up this article out of his head, was incompetent in researching the literature, or had a sincere desire to protect the American people from a disease about which he was totally ignorant.

Irresponsible, incompetent, malicious-too strong? Harris admits to J. Howard Brown of Johns Hopkins University that he made the whole thing up and from his own writings reveals that he knew it couldn't have possibly happened.

A Summary of Harris' "Facts"

1) Undulant fever is a common disease in the United States. *Untrue*

2) Raw milk transmits undulant fever. *Untrue*

3) Cows that have passed tests for undulant fever can pass the germ in their milk. *Untrue*

4) Cows can transmit the pig strain of undulant fever in their milk. *Untrue*

5) Undulant fever can be transmitted from cheese. *Untrue*

6) Four thousand cases of typhoid fever in Montreal were caused by drinking raw milk. *Untrue* (It was pasteurized milk.

7) Drinking unpasteurized milk unnecessarily exposes one to illness. *Untrue*

8) Ten percent of Americans are infected with undulant fever. *Untrue* (And preposterous!)

9) Raw milk can be "as lethal as strychnine." *Untrue* (And asinine.)

Americans believe in the Reader's Digest and Ladies Home Journal and, for the most part, in my opinion, this trust is justified. J.B. Darlington, in her brilliant series of articles in the *Rural New Yorker*, remarks that a free press, such as we have, would appear to guarantee that both sides will be heard on an issue. If, such as in the case of raw milk, articles appear in prestigious journals like the Reader's Digest and Ladies Home Journal attacking raw milk as unsafe and no reply is heard in future issues, then unpasteurized milk stands convicted. After all, we have a free press.

But a "free press" is free to print or not print, so it will print what is in the best interest of the press. The best interest of the press coincides with the interest of its advertisers. In the dairy industry, close to one hundred percent of the advertising is done by the National Dairy Council and those closely affiliated with it. They do not consider raw milk to be in their best financial interest and, hence, the American people have been subjected to a one-sided propaganda blast that depicts fresh, unpasteurized milk as a veritable bacterial soup and a sure path to an early grave. Pasteurization has been sold as a cure-all, and the people, after years of propaganda, have accepted it as being as true as the law of gravity. The press is not free for everyone, and Coronet refused to allow the other side of the milk controversy to be heard.

The Ladies Home Journal, December, 1944, reported, "A Kansas City survey proved that nine percent of 7,122 school children entertained (undulant fever) infection."

"Entertained," a peculiar word in this context, could be interpreted by most people as meaning that almost seven hundred children of those surveyed were running around with undulant fever-an epidemic.

Darlington *(Rural New Yorker)* investigated this claim. Both Kansas City, Missouri and Kansas City, Kansas health departments denied any knowledge of the survey. After further research, Darlington finally found the report that the Kansas Cities had no knowledge of.

The report did indeed reveal nine percent-but nine percent of what? The study merely showed that nine percent of the children had a positive skin test to brucellosis, like a TB skin test, but *not a single case of undulant fever was found.* Not only were the children not "entertaining the infection" as reported by Ladies Home Journal, but, because of their positive skin tests, which indicate immunity, *it would be almost impossible for them to contract the disease.*

The pasteurization propagandists will use the flimsiest statistics in their relentless drive to stamp out raw milk. The Progressive, on July 15, 1946 and repeated by the Reader's Digest the following month, reported:

> "Startling improvements in public health invariably ensue when a community moves from raw to pasteurized milk. The Province of Ontario, Canada had been overrun with undulant fever, typhoid, and other infectious diseases when, in 1938, the provincial legislature made pasteurization compulsory in all communities ...deaths from typhoid were cut in half."

As we pointed out in our analysis of the Coronet article, whether milk is pasteurized or not has little to do with catching typhoid. But the most impressive thing about the author of this propaganda piece is not his ignorance, but his audacity. The official records from the Canadian Public Health Journal and the Ontario Department of Health reveal that between 1912 and 1941 inclusive, a period of twenty-nine years, there was a grand total of two deaths from milk-borne typhoid. Cut in half? From two to one in twenty-nine years? Although the statistics don't tell us, there is a good possibility that the milk involved was pasteurized anyway.

The other typhoid deaths during this period, two hundred forty-five of them, were caused by contaminated foods other than milk and just plain water. From these statistics it becomes obvious that milk is one of the foods *least likely* to give you typhoid fever.

The Reader's Digest, enlarging on the Progressive's hysterical and dishonest article, reported:

> "...an estimated 45,000 persons will be stricken this year with one or another of the lethal diseases carried by infected raw milk-diseases such as diphtheria, streptococcus infections of the throat and tonsils, dysentery, scarlet, typhoid, paratyphoid, and undulant fever. Still more thousands will suffer debilitating gastric and intestinal disturbances which are likely to be put down to 'food poisoning'. Thousands of infants will contract diarrhea, more or less serious."

Wow, our old friend the cow is nothing but a four-legged Typhoid Mary!

But, knowing the old adage about statistics and statisticians, we looked at the records for the years 1944 and 1945, which are the two years preceding the Progressive article and the Reader's Digest condensation.

Official public health reports for those two years reveal:

Diseases from raw milk and raw milk in ice cream	904 cases
Diseases from pasteurized milk and pasteurized milk in ice cream	1,841 cases

Darlington (The Rural New Yorker), to emphasize the relative unimportance of milk in transmitting disease, gives the following comparisons for the year 1944:

Diseases from milk and milk products 1,499 cases

Diseases from water   2,686 cases

Diseases from foods other than milk   14,558 cases

Raw milk accounted for a little over two percent of this total and Darlington comments wryly, "If evidence to support the promotion of pasteurization is so difficult to find that it must needs be distorted and in some cases even invented . . . an honest mind cannot fail to grasp that the case for pasteurization is a very weak case indeed."

The propaganda blitz in the lay press has, unfortunately, been supported by the majority of professional organizations.

The opposition to unprocessed raw milk includes:

American Veterinary Medical Association
American Medical Association
American Dental Association
American Academy of Pediatrics
Federal Food and Drug Administration
Center for Disease Control
National Dairy Council
State and county health departments
U.S. Animal Health Association
National Association of State Public Health
      Veterinarians
Conference of State and Territorial Epidemiologists

With this kind of opposition, the tiny group of dairymen producing top quality, untreated milk can survive only if the American consumer educates himself about milk and then, in turn, enlists the aid of his doctor and his state legislators. As the people responsible for the nation's health are largely misinformed on the subject of milk, the impetus for the return to healthy milk must come from the consumer.

This relentless propaganda has reduced the number of raw certified dairies to three: Two in California and one in Georgia. Public health officials and misinformed professional groups across the country continue their vicious attacks against the three remaining raw certified milk producers.

A recent anti-milk book,[10] *Don't Drink Your Milk* by Oski, brought up the old argument about other mammals not drinking milk after weaning. Man is the only mammal, the argument goes, who drinks milk after the weaning age. Therefore it is abnormal and against nature's intent.

But man is one of the few mammals who eats snails, raw clams, and raw oysters. He is the only mammal who eats lobster. Most mammals are restricted in what they eat by their ecological circumstances. They can only eat what nature provides. Man, with his mobility and intelligence, has a wide variety of foods to choose from.* Most mammals, if offered fresh milk, will drink it and like it. Try it on your cat.

Oski's anti-milk book implicates milk in a wide range of diseases including anemia, arthritis, "Lou Gehrig Disease," fatigue, allergy, and multiple sclerosis. But, tragically, the author didn't understand that man, not the cow, is the culprit and that pasteurization and homogenization** cause most of the ills he blames on milk. Arthritis and multiple sclerosis, two of the diseases he blames on milk, can actually be treated with raw milk (See Chapter XI).

---

* Granted, he doesn't always make a wise choice.

** He doesn't even mention homogenization.

Oski's book does contain an excellent chapter on the politics of milk. Since he wrote his book, the political situation has gotten much worse. President Reagan, who is supposed to be a conservative, signed into law a bill that pays dairy farmers not to produce milk. So the dairy farmer, like the potato farmer, joins a privileged class paid not to work. Udderly disgusting.*

THE GREAT SALMONELLA
FISH STORY

Salmonella is not a fish but a form of bacteria. But public health officials and the scientists who should know better, act awfully fishy about salmonella. If you don't understand salmonella you won't understand the Alta-Dena conspiracy that follows. Once you understand the basic bacteriology of milk** you will see how incredible the conspiracy against Alta-Dena and Mathis Dairies really is.

The organism was named after the American veterinarian, D.E. Salmon, who isolated it in 1885. It is ubiquitous. Salmonella is in your nose; it is in the living room rug. There is salmonella in your gut and plenty in your hair. Your cat has it too.*** *It is also in your food-all of your food that hasn't been sterilized and sealed in a container.*

A CDC report in 1978 revealed that meat was far and away the most common cause of salmonella food poisoning. Other causes were mayonnaise, water, Mexican food, potato salad, hamburger casserole, and tacos. So what's all this stuff about milk? Even Peruvian fish meal and turtles have caused salmonella food poisoning but raw certified milk?—Never.

---

* Where do I sign up for a double dip? I'll promise not to practice medicine or write books.

** There will be no written examination.

*** As high as 40% in some cat populations.[9]

Another common source of salmonella poisoning is cheese *from pasteurized milk.* One epidemic in Colorado' put three hundred thirty-nine people in the outhouse. There were no fatalities, but everyone got their intestinal tract thoroughly scoured. The CDC reported[2] an outbreak of salmonella food poisoning in Arizona. Twenty-three people sick-from *pasteurized* milk. An epidemic in Ohio was caused by marijuana. The smokers then transmitted it to their children and the children infected their grandmothers.*

The CDC appears to be as eager as the California Health Department to stamp out raw certified milk. They supported the California Health Services vicious and unwarranted attacks against Alta-Dena. They editorialized, ". . . salmonella contamination of unpasteurized milk can be a persistent problem, *even in dairies that follow the procedures recommended by the American Association of Medical Milk Commissions...*"** (Emphasis added.) They concluded, "Present day technology cannot produce raw milk (including that listed as certified) that can be assured to be free of pathogens; only with pasteurization is there this assurance." You might expect that sort of statement from a high school biology report, but not from the Ph.D's, M.D.'s and vets at the Center for Disease Control. Actually, "present day technology" solved the problem years ago with the introduction of the automatic milk machine.

Another illustration of the CDC's competence level was a July, 1977 report[3] in which they state that Q Fever can be caught from raw milk. Q Fever has never been contracted from drinking milk, raw or pasteurized. The disease comes only from inhaling the organisms.***

In October, 1978 there was an epidemic of salmonella food poisoning in Arizona[4] involving sixty-six peo-

---

* Will the FDA require the pasteurization of marijuana?

** How can I say this delicately? That's a plain damn lie.

*** One research group claims to have proven that Q Fever can be transmitted through milk. Their work was not convincing.

ple which was caused by pasteurized milk. The bacteria level was *twenty-three times the legal limit and the CDC reported that the milk had been properly pasteurized.* The pasteurization had nothing to do with it. If that milk had not been pasteurized, raw milk that is, lack of pasteurization would have been blamed for the epidemic. Yet the Center for Disease Control continues to tell us that, "... only with pasteurization is there... assurance" against infection.*

The CDC undertook to tell sanitarians "what they should know" about salmonella in 1967. An article appeared in a technical milk journal in December, and three months later, March, 1968, the same material reappeared in the Journal of the American Medical Association. The first article blamed salmonella contamination of powdered milk on raw milk from *one cow* out of *eight hundred* dairy farms. As this particular plant handles *eleven million pounds* of milk every year from tens of thousands of cows, it would be statistically impossible for one cow to be responsible. Even if one cow were heavily infected, the dilutive factor makes this supposition ridiculous.

What was not mentioned in the first article was brought out in the second one. Two workers in the plant were found to be infected with salmonella. As usual, raw milk got the blame. They can heat the milk all day, and if there are dirty workers at the packaging end of the line, the salmonella will be in the packaged milk.

The CDC, again backing up the hit men of the California Department of Health, reported[5] that Alta-Dena raw milk "has been implicated in outbreaks of salmonella in 1958, 1964, and 1971-1975." This was proven to be absolutely false.** The staff veterinarian of the Iowa De-

---

* The CDC doesn't seem to understand. You can't pasteurize the people who handle our food. But if food handlers were checked more vigorously than the food, most epidemics could be eliminated.

** !%(x!/o bureaucrats.

partment of Health repeated the California falsehoods to justify the compulsory pasteurization of milk in Iowa. They embellished on California's phony reports and struck fear into the raw milk drinkers by stating that raw certified milk cannot be guaranteed free from disease because the salmonella germs are shed intermittently into the milk from the cow's blood.[6] Not so.

Iowa doesn't stop at just scaring the bejesus out of its citizens concerning raw milk. They don't fool around. The Iowa courts have ruled that "it is within the scope of the *police power* to require . . . that all milk for human consumption must be pasteurized." Now that's dedication.

The most recent attack against raw (and pasteurized) milk is the leukemia reports.[7] Some cows do indeed have a leukemia called Bovine Leukemia Virus (BLV). But human blood studies have *never* shown the presence of the virus. Millions of Americans have been raised on raw milk, yet leukemia is not a common disease. In India almost all of the milk is unpasteurized, but leukemia is not a common disease there either-another bum rap against milk.

Not all state health departments are as ignorant as those in California, Nevada, and Iowa. A letter from the Pennsylvania Bureau of Foods and Chemistry~ left no doubt about their confidence in raw milk, "I can think of no incident in Pennsylvania in the past twenty years in which raw milk was determined to have been the cause of human illness."

The California Health Department, apparently unable to sell its shabby research in the United States, took its road show to England and got it published in the British Medical Journal. They reported that "Dairy X" (Alta-Dena Dairy of California) was wiping out poor cancer patients with their infernal raw milk contaminated with salmonella. Two Scottish experts responded, in essence, that the California Health Department was blowing smoke, "...we found no evidence of... life-threatening potential on the part of salmonella..." They had examined *seven hundred cases* in England without finding a single really serious case.

The three courageous certified dairies producing raw certified milk are a highly select group of farmers with a desire to supply the people with clean, nutritious milk. Health departments are expending their time and taxpayers money pursuing a problem where none exists.* It is ironic that health bureaucrats over-inspect the milk producers who are least likely to have milk contaminated with salmonella or any other bacteria. I stated in testimony before the California Milk Commission, the group responsible for milk sanitation in California, that looking for salmonella at the Alta-Dena Certified Dairy or the Mathis Certified Dairy in Georgia is like looking for atheists in a Baptist church. You might find one occasionally, but your yield would be extremely low.

If you want to find salmonella, go where the action is. Go to commercial food establishments, barbecues, church socials. Check the mayonnaise, roast beef, and the custard pie. Forget the raw certified milk. It's the *one* food that you know is okay.

To bring you up to date, Vogue Magazine of July, 1984, blasted raw milk. Their health section was headlined: RAW-MILK WARNING.**

"A new and dangerous fad: drinking raw or certified raw milk, also known as unpasteurized milk. In a recent newsletter of the California Council Against Health Frauds, John Bolton, M.D., cautions that people drinking raw milk are at increased risk of salmonella infection, which can result in high fevers and bloody diarrhea. In 1983, the risk of contracting salmonella was 118 times

---

* That's not unusual for bureaucrats.

** I don't know why they hyphenated raw milk. Like murder suicide I guess.

greater for those who drank raw milk than for those who did not."

That statement, as pointed out in the next chapter, is based on misusing statistics. The years reported for those statistics in Chapter IV were 1944 and 1945, but nothing has changed, and they are still lying about raw milk, using invalid statistics compiled by medical bureaucrats.

Why are the state health departments so fanatical and malicious toward the raw milk dealers? Part of the answer is undoubtedly ignorance of the scientific facts. Give the average health officer (or doctor) a quiz on the infectious aspects of raw versus pasteurized milk and the nutritional differences between them, and he will most likely flunk.

But an equally important reason is the economic one. Professor Oscar Erf pointed this out over forty years ago,[9] "The Board of Health and cities, as a rule, are unwilling to spend money for this inspection (of raw milk) to secure a good nutritious milk supply to those who want it. *This is where the difficulty usually lies.*"

State officials resorted to outright deception of the public to discredit raw milk in South Carolina. I testified before the South Carolina legislature on raw milk, and I was astounded at the sneaky methods used by the state and university officials in the attempt to discredit raw milk.

State veterinarian, C.E. Boyd, told the horror story of a herd of 385 dairy cows that he had destroyed because half of them were "tuberculosis reactive". Boyd knew perfectly well that a positive skin test for TB, a "tuberculosis reactor," did not mean the reactor had tuberculosis. Ninety-nine percent of the time it means that the animal (or person) is immune to tuberculosis.

I testified that half of the hundred people in the hearing room undoubtedly had positive skin tests for tuberculosis, but that did not mean they had to be slaughtered or even treated. Even if the cows had TB, I said, the milk would still be okay to drink. I pointed out that tuberculous *people*, not cows or cow's milk, give tuberculosis to people.

Intestinal TB used to be caused by tubercular milk. This was caused by a tubercular milker hacking into the milk pail, flies or other insects and contamination by manure. All of this has been eliminated by closed system automatic milking machines. And, as Dr. Boyd knows, it is extremely rare to find a cow today with active tuberculosis anyway.

To illustrate how scientists can manipulate the people's representatives and how the press can manipulate the rest of us, we reproduce below an editorial that appeared in the Columbia, South Carolina Record following the Senate hearing.*

The Columbia Record
PUBLISHED BY COLUMBIA NEWSPAPERS, INC.
Afternoon Newspaper Established in 1897 in Columbia, South Carolina
8-A   Tuesday, April 27, 1982 **RECORD'S EDITORIALS**
Nay To Raw Milk

While we'd hoped that a bill to allow commercial production of unpasteurized milk in South Carolina would languish away in the Senate's Medical Affairs Committee, such was not to be. Unfortunate.

However, Sen. Hyman Rubin, who heads the committee, said he was bringing the bill onto the calendar "out of fairness" to Sen. T. Ed Garrison of Anderson. A dairy farmer and chairman of the Agriculture Committee, Garrison is a chief advocate of the measure.

Rubin is personally opposed. We're on Rubin's side– against.

We trust that the bill will sour, spoil and be tossed away as it's stacked with other bills on the Senate calendar shelves. No cold storage.

Should the bill go before the Senate, we trust that senators will recall testimony of leading medical men and Dr. Robert L. Jackson, DHEC commissioner.

Jackson says, "It's not possible for any inspection or regulation to ensure that raw milk is as safe as pasteurized milk.

---

* The other half of the story, my testimony and that of Mr. Jack Mathis of the Mathis Dairy, Atlanta, Georgia was ignored.

I'm opposed to the bill because continued pasteurization is the only way we can ensure a safe milk product." Right as rain.

Jackson cited, and senators should always remember, 22 cases and two deaths from salmonella connected with raw milk consumption in the state of Washington last year. Another item: 260 raw milk-related products endangered citizens of Kansas last year.

Chilling, indeed, is the testimony of *C.E. Boyd, state veterinarian.* Consider his credentials: he's director of the Clemson University Livestock-Poultry Health Depart-

ment. He told the story of a herd of 385 dairy cows that had to be "depopulated" when more than half were found to be *tuberculosis reactors.* Milk from those sickly cows was pasteurized before being marketed.

"I can't predict what would have happened if that milk had been sold raw."

Allow commercial production of unpasteurized milk in our state? Give us one vote and we'll shout "Nay!" Give us two votes and you have "Nay, Nay!" Give us three and hear: "Nay, Nay, Nay!" (Emphasis added.)

THE TROJAN COW

The Medical Milk Commission, responsible for certifying as to the purity of milk, had taken a strong stand against pasteurization since their inception at the turn of the 20th century. They defended clean unpasteurized milk, properly inspected, as the milk of choice because of its superior nutrition, better digestibility, and freedom from disease-causing properties suspected of being in heated milk.

But in 1929 the camel got his nose in the tent. In September of that year, the first pasteurized certified milk was sold. There was vigorous objection to this from members of the milk commission and producers of raw certified milk. Certification, they said, was for the purpose of guaranteeing disease-free milk, making the destructive process of pasteurization unnecessary. The issue would become blurred and confused. The consumer would come to think, erroneously, that pasteurization was an added benefit to certification of the raw product.

But why have raw milk *at all* if the pasteurized milk is certified as to purity? The whole purpose of raw certified milk, the avoidance of the destructive pasteurization process, while at the same time producing pure milk, was being subverted. A member of the milk commission said, "It is at times distressing to see forces at work trying to eliminate or destroy our cause. More effort is expended to accomplish this end than trying to do something about the sixty percent of milk that remains unprotected, even by pasteurization."

A major factor in the demise of the raw certified milk industry was World War II. Milk could not be shipped halfway around the world in its natural state. This gave a great impetus to pasteurization and powdered pasteurized milk.

A near fatal blow was dealt to the raw certified milk producers by the hiring of Mr. Charles Speakes as Secretary-Treasurer of the American Association of Medical Milk Commissions, the national organization responsible for maintaining the standards, educating the public, and encouraging milk producers to produce raw certified milk. Speakes was a double agent. Unbeknownst to the Milk Commission, he was also the Executive Secretary of the Milk Foundation-which is dedicated to the eradication of raw milk, certified or otherwise!

By the time the raw milk producers realized that they were being subverted from the inside, the battle was practically over. When Mr. Jack Mathis, President of Mathis Dairy in Atlanta, went to Washington to fire Speakes, he found two telephones on his desk, one for the Milk Commission and one for the Milk Foundation. "We never had a chance," Mathis remarked sadly.

With the firing of Speakes, the official journal, Certified Milk Magazine, ceased to exist. The magazine had served the raw certified milk industry for forty years, but it had become, under Speakes, an impotent publication no longer defending or even advocating raw certified milk. In the 30's raw certified milk was vigorously defended in the pages of Certified Milk Magazine. After Speakes took over the editorship, the word "raw" was rarely mentioned. Fresh, unprocessed milk was a dead issue, defeated by a Trojan cow.

REFERENCES

1. American Journal of Epidemiology, Volume III, Nr.2, pp.247.

2. MMWR, March 16, 1979.

3. Ibid., July 22, 1977.

4. Ibid., March 16, 1979.

5. Ibid., March 1, 1981.

6. Iowa Department of Health letter, February 20,1981.

7. McClure, et al, Cancer Research, 34:2745-2757, 1974.

8. Private communication, August 9, 1979.

9. History of Randleigh Farms, pp.255.

10. JAMA, February 12, 1982, pp. 816.

11. Don't Drink Your Milk, Oski and Bell, Wyden Books, 1977.

Chapter V

A COW IS NOT A CAT–
"CERTIFIED" MILK

This chapter is "R" rated. If you don't like words like s--t, skip over to page 64.

There's one thing you have got to understand. A cow is not a cat. A cat can't *stand* to be dirty. They don't even like to get their feet wet. But a cow just doesn't give a damn. They will defecate where they sleep. They will defecate where they eat. They stand in it and they will lie in it. Their legs, udders, and often even their necks are splattered with a combination of mud and cow shit.* Cows are not neat. Their personal hygiene would embarrass a pig.** Cows are loveable at a distance-and downwind.

Cows produce a lot of two things. One of them is milk. But milk production is in second place to the main product of the cow which is cow manure. Unfortunately, many dairies bottle a product which is a combination of item one and item two.

In the course of my research, I visited dozens of dairies, and I was appalled at the lack of hygiene in handling the cows. The uncertified dairies often milk cows with manure heavily coated on the hind legs. The milk suction tubes can easily rub against these filthy areas. The teats are supposed to be carefully wiped off before

---

* Hold your nose and read it anyway. You really need to keep abreast of what's going on down on the farm.

** A pig will not poop in his parlor. If he can't get out, he will at least go in the corner.

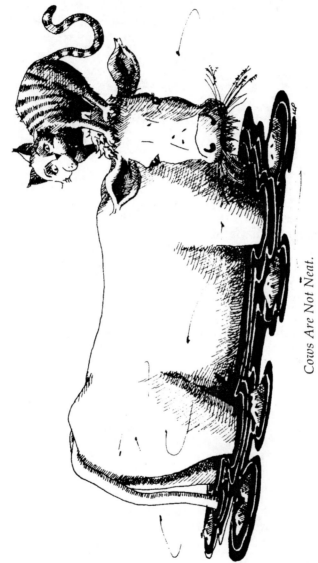

Cows Are Not Neat.

milking. In poorly supervised operations, the milker carries a paper towel in the back pocket of his jeans. Sometimes he wipes off the teats, and sometimes he doesn't. This procedure is extremely important because the hose-spraying of the teats, which is universally used, only removes the obvious debris. As you know from cleaning your car, spraying the surface with a hose is not effective. You must wipe away the surface dirt. The same is true of a cow teat.

This was demonstrated to me quite dramatically at the Alta-Dena Dairy in Chino, California. Paul Virgin, my tour guide and good friend, took a hose and sprayed the teats of a cow in the usual manner. He then took a white towel from the stack and wiped one of the four teats— *plenty* of mud and manure on the towel. If those teats aren't cleaned properly, and they often are not, *that stuff goes in your milk.* Sure, they pasteurize it. But do you want pus, feces, mud, and urine from the neighboring goat in your milk even if it has been heated?

After visiting these dairies and comparing them to Alta-Dena in California and Mathis in Georgia, I will *never* drink any milk but raw certified milk. To produce certified milk, the teats and udders must be properly cleaned. Alta-Dena uses *twenty thousand* white towels a day cleaning udders. The Brand X dairies use paper kitchen "towels" when they use anything at all. They may use one paper towel on as many as six cows.* Alta-Dena and Mathis use 1-1/2 towels per cow.

Why does the dairy industry resist producing raw certified milk in the light of all the evidence proving that homogenized, pasteurized milk is an inferior, unhealthy food? Look at the following comparison between raw certified and pasteurized milk and you will see why. It takes dedication to cleanliness, time, and money to produce good milk.

Don't stop. This stuff is important. I know you're not a scientist, but your family's health is involved here-read

---

*I counted.

on. If you just can't *stand* tables, at least read 1), 2), 6), 7), 8), 11), 13), 17), 19), 20), 24), and 25).

It would be embarrassing to the producers of junk milk ("Grade A Pasteurized, Vitamin D Milk") if the consumers found out about these differences. How could the junk milk producers live with these purists? What would it do to their profits? Wouldn't they look shoddy and irresponsible?

So they went to their best defense, the Big Lie, "All raw milk is unsafe." This being true, we must pasteurize it for the safety of the consumer. What the consumer didn't know was that milk so filthy that it has to be pasteurized to make it safe to drink is certainly *dangerous* when raw and unhealthy when pasteurized.

Patricia R. Meyer did an exhaustive study of the certified milk industry. She concluded: *"Raw certified milk is unique in that it is the only significant source of a complete food in our diet that is not processed in some form before being eaten.*

"It is only appropriate that consumers have singled out this food as an issue involving their choice to buy food and weigh the risk/benefit concept themselves. Some of the claims for raw certified milk may never be scientifically proven and some already have. Raw certified milk, although a minor factor quantitatively in our food market, is an outstanding example of the epitomy of the highest quality of food that man has available. In every sense it is a product that speaks for itself. From all indications, it is here to stay. The specific conclusions arrived at from this work include:

1) When methods and standards for raw certified milk production are considered, risk of contracting disease from its consumption is highly unlikely.
2) Raw certified milk is respected by certified milk customers because it is one of the few highly nutritious foods available that has not been processed.

Category Compared	Raw Certified Milk	Pasteurized Milk
1) Enzymes:	All available.	Less than 10% remaining.
2) Protein:	100% available, all 22 amino acids, including 8 that are essential.	Protein-lysine and tyrosine are altered by heat with serious loss of metabolic availability. This results in making the whole protein complex less available for tissue repair and rebuilding.
3) Fats: (research studies indicate that fats are necessary to metabolize protein and calcium. All natural protein-bearing foods contain fats.)	All 18 fatty acids metabolically available, both saturated and unsaturated fats.	Altered by heat, especially the 10 essential unsaturated fats.
4) Vitamins:	All 100% available.	Among the fat-soluble vitamins, some are classed as unstable and therefore a loss is caused by heating above blood temperature. This loss can run as high as 66%. Vitamin C loss usually exceeds 50%. Losses on water-soluble vitamins are affected by heat and can run from 38%7o to 80%.

5) Carbohydrates:	Easily utilized in metabolism. Still associated naturally with elements.	Tests indicate that heat has made some changes making elements less available metabolically.
6) Minerals:	All 100% metabolically available. Major mineral components are calcium, chlorine, magnesium, phosphorus, potassium, sodium and sulphur. Vital trace minerals, all 24 or more, 100% available.	Calcium is altered by heat and loss in metabolism may run 50% or more, depending on pasteurization temperature. Losses in other essential minerals, because one mineral usually acts as a synergistic for another element. There is a loss of enzymes that serve as leaders in assimilation minerals.
7) Cleanliness:	Milk tested daily at an independent laboratory for the Certified Milk Commission in all states.	Never tested over twice per month by the Department of Health.
8) Bacteria count for standard plate count:		
Milk:	10,000/milliliter maximum at all certified dairies.	In Georgia 100,000/ml before pasteurization and 30,000 after. In New York 100,000 before and 30,000 after pasteurization. In California 75,000/ml maximUm before pasteurization and 15,000 after. 25,000/ml maximum.
Cream:	10,000/ml maximum in all states.	
9) Anaerobic bacteria test	Once a week in all states.	None required in any state.°

° You can test for these bacteria in your milk. See Appendix II.

Category Compared	Raw Certified Milk	Pasteurized Milk
10) Streptococci:	Once a month in all states.	None required in any state.
11) Herd tests:	Each cow is blood tested for brucellosis before entering the milk herd and receives a blood test at least once a year. Reactors are removed at all certified dairies.	Blood tests are made on a herd only if ring tests on milk are questionable. Reactors are removed in all states.
	All dairy cows in certified herds are vaccinated for brucellosis between the age of 4 - 6 months.	*Not all cows are vaccinated.*
12) T.B. skin test:	*Every 180 days* by a state veterinarian.	Tested annually.
13) Sanitarian visits:	Once a month, from the Certified Milk Commission at all certified dairies.	No visits required in most states.
14) Employee Health Examinations:	All new employees have a complete physical; plus monthly exams of each employee thereafter at all certified dairies.	Routine examination required at time of employment in some states.

15) Streptococcus throat culture:	Monthly in all states for employees.	Not required for employees.
16) Chest X-ray:	Yearly in all states for employees.	Not required for employees.
17) Stool specimen:	Twice a year in all states for employees.	Not required for employees.
18) Keeping Qualities:	Bacteria growth in Certified Milk increases very slowly because friendly acid-forming bacteria (nature's antiseptic retards the growth of invading organisms—bacteria). Cerdfied Raw Milk, produced clean and not exposed to air or human touch, usually keeps for two weeks under constant refrigeration and later will sour.	Bacteria growth in pasteurized milk (minimum pasteurization temp. usually is 161° for 18 sec.) will be geometric (rapid). After pasteurizing and homogenizing, milk gradually turns rancid but never will sour. Rancid milk is not palatable.
19) Health of the cows:	Examined once a month by a veterinarian designated by the County Milk Commission.	Not required.
	General health of the milking herd is checked.	Not required.
	Reproductive tract of each cow that has freshened is examined and treated if necessary. Condition and treatments are recorded for future reference.	Not required.

Category Compared	Raw Certified Milk	Pasteurized Milk
	All heifer calves must be vaccinated for brucellosis between 3-5 months of age.	No heifer vaccination required.
	Herds shall be tested for tuberculosis every 6 months.	Once every 6 years.
	A monthly CMT test shall be performed on the milk of all lactating cows. Milk from cows showing a 500,000 cells/ml. or higher reaction will be cultured on a blood agar plate for evidence of pathogenic organisms. A positive pathogen test will automatically remove a cow from the milking line. Such cows shall be checked and certified to be free of pathogenic organisms before returning to the milking line.	Leucocyte count may not exceed 1,500,000 per ml. Bulk tank milk is checked 8 times a year. Cultures on individual cows not required.
	Bacterial check on all quarters (teats) following delivery of calf	Not required.

	A blood agar plate culture of all quarters shall be made on each cow within 10 days of being turned dry. Quarters harboring any pathogenic bacteria will be treated with appropriate antibiotics during the dry period.	Not required.
20) Milking Procedure:	The udder and teats shall be washed, sanitized, and dried immediately prior to milking.	Must be milked under "sanitary conditions." *Sanitizing of udder not required.*
	Each quarter at every milking shall be examined for detection of abnormal milk prior to the application of the milking machine.	Not required.
	Following removal of the milking machine, each teat shallbe immersed or sprayed with an approved teat-dip bacteriocide.	Not required.
21) Milking Equipment:	All milking equipment-glass, stainless steel, or rubber that comes in contact with certified milk shall be cleaned and sanitized before and after milking. The cleaning solution must be at least 140° F. and must be circulated for a minimum of 20 min.	"Milk must be produced under sanitary conditions."

Category Compared	Raw Certified Milk	Pasteurized Milk
	Milking equipment will be designed and installed to minimize flooding from the teat end of the receiver jar. To facilitate this, the following items are suggested: 1) air valves in liner; 2) alternate pulsations; 3) large—at least 2"—low level milk line; 4) vaccuum pump capacity of at least 20 CFM(N.Z.) per milker unit; 5) all vacuum levels should not exceed 12"13" during milking operations.	Not required.
	Alternate teat cup rubber inflations after 350 milkings or 7 days, whichever comes first.	Not required.
	The rubber inflations shall be replaced after 700 milkings.	Not required.
22) Milk Quality:	Maximum allowable bacteria per milliliter of milk—10,000.	Generally tested 4 times each 6 months by the health department.

	Maximum allowable coliform bacteria per milliliter of milk—10.	Bacteria—Maximum count 100,000 per ml. before pasteurization; 20,000 per ml. maximum after. Not exceeding 300,000 per ml as commingled milk prior to pasteurization.
		Coliform bacteria count not checked on raw, but cannot exceed 10 per ml after pasteurization.
	Milk is considered of excellent quality when the concentration of leucocytes does not exceed *500,000 per ml.*	Leucocyte count may not exceed *1,500,000 per ml.*
23) Cooling:	Milk must be cooled to 40° F. within one hour after completion of milking and maintained at this temperature until delivered to the consumer.	Cool to 50° or less and maintain thereat until processed.
24) Housing:	Free stalls or equal facilities shall be required for a herd used to produce certified milk. Bedding must be dry and maintained daily. Feeding areas, loafing areas, etc., must be scraped, cleaned, and disinfected daily.	No specific regulation.

Category Compared	Raw Certified Milk	Pasteurized Milk
25) Visitors:	Visitors coming from other areas where livestock were present on the premises shall be required to wear plastic boots or other approved shoe covers while present on the farm.	Not required.
26) Employee Health Examinations:	All new employees have complete physical examinauon and tests when starting to work on a certified farm.	Not required.
	Every 180 days each farm employee who milks cows must have required medical tests.	Not required.
	It will be the duty of every employee who milks cows to report immediately any illness he may have to his superintendent.	Not required.

NOTE:

Bacteria growth in Certified Raw Milk increases very slowly, for the friendly acid-forming bacteria (nature's antiseptic) retards the growth of invading organisms (bacteria).

a) Usually keeps for several weeks when under constant refrigeration and will sour.

b) Produced clean and not exposed to air or human touch.

*

_____
*Wasn't that interesting?

Pasteurization refers to the process of heating every particle of milk to at least 145° F. and holding at such temperature for at least 15 seconds. Pasteurizing does not remove dirt, dead bacterially-produced toxins from milk. Bacteria growth will be geometrically rapid after pasteurizing and homogenizing. Milk gradually turns rancid in a few days, and then decomposes.

3) Consumers of raw certified milk are very concerned about the premium price they must pay for this milk, but remain staunchly willing to do so.

4) There may be an inherent factor in raw certified milk that permits people who are allergic to pasteurized cow milk to drink raw certified milk without adverse effects.

5) There is a statistically significant higher value of some of the water soluable vitamins in raw certified milk than in pasteurized milk.

6) Sales of raw certified milk are restricted by legalities in fourteen states and by the lack of certified dairies in the United States. These factors would have to be changed before full-scale distribution could be achieved.

7) Further experimentation to prove or disprove some of the claims made for certified milk should be completed.*

To give some idea of the stringency with which the Milk Commission controls the potential bacterial contamination in raw certified milk, let's look at one of the regulations of the Milk Commission. A potential danger from milk (as with many foods) is bacterial hemolytic streptococcus. The streptococcus can cause strep throat and scarlet fever. The regulations state, "If any cow should be found to harbor Group A, hemolytic streptococci, she shall be *immediately* and *permanently* removed from the herd."

A great deal has been made of the difference of the flavor of pasteurized homogenized milk as compared to raw milk. Some people simply do not like the taste of raw milk because it's not what they are accustomed to. The devotees of raw certified milk say that it is far more

---

*Now go back to page 66 and read the table.

delicious; in fact, the children of these people will generally prefer raw milk. It's interesting to note that the regulations concerning raw milk as put out by the Medical
Milk Commission states, "The flavor of milk is closely associated with its nutritional value. The methods outlined
for producing milk of high nutritional value are also important for producing the best milk flavor."

In 192 5 Dr. Paul B. Cassidy lamented publicly that
the majority of doctors were abandoning raw milk for babies in favor of evaporated, condensed, or powdered
milk. He was a great supporter of raw certified milk and
was at one time the secretary of the American Association of Medical Milk Commissions. The AAMMC is the
group of doctors responsible for seeing that the dairies
carrying the certification seal stay up to the standards of
cleanliness required by the milk commission.

Cassidy reported before a dairy convention[2] the phenomenal results he had had at St. Vincent's Hospital in
Philadelphia by switching from pasteurized to raw certified milk. The commercial pasteurized milk often had a
bacteria count of 200,000.* The sister in charge of the hospital was very concerned about the high death among infants from gastroenteritis. She asked Dr. Cassidy for his
advice, and he recommended a switch from pasteurized
to raw certified milk.

The pasteurization Chicken Littles predicted that
there would be a catastrophic increase in infant deaths
from using raw milk. The death rate from gastroenteritis
quickly fell from a high of 89 in 1922 to less than five per
year.

Emily Bacon, a pioneer woman doctor, was enthusiastic about raw certified milk and urged its use, especially for babies and growing children, "It is the best milk
for infants and growing children because it is clean, it is
safe, it is raw, it is uniform in consistency, it is fresh. Its
safety is assured because it is Certified Milk... there are

---

*And still does.

no harmful bacteria in it. *Because it is safe, it does not need to be pasteurized."*

A remarkable quality of milk that housewives of pioneer days in the West took advantage of was its ability to preserve meat. The resourceful housewives would immerse chops, steaks and roasts in large crocks of buttermilk, thus assuring fresh meat for the family year round.

The Arabs have been preserving meat with camel milk for thousands of years. The Icelanders of 200 years ago preserved their sheep's heads in sour milk.[3]

In 1908, an American doctor decided to try it himself. He immersed a beefsteak in buttermilk. *Thirteen years later* it was in a state of perfect preservation, "showing not the slightest taint or decay."

The doctor emphasized that only raw milk could be used for this preservative effect, "It should be mentioned right here; however, that these remarks are true only of clean cow's milk as it flows from the original fount, and do not hold for milk which has been boiled or pasteurized... processes which... deprive the milk of one of its most unique and valuable properties."[4]

Raw certified milk was extremely popular among leaders in medicine before World War II. The prestigious Hartford Hospital used only certified milk, most of it raw, "in the artificial feeding of infants, for expectant and nursing mothers, *and for all other cases."*

Harris Moak, M.D., a well-respected physician of the early 20th century, made statements that sound a little depressing as we near the end of that century. He asked rhetorically, "Does it seem at all likely that public health officials, the great majority of whom are Doctors of Medicine as well as Doctors of Public Health, will ever deny their brothers in the medical profession the right to have clean, pure, thoroughly trustworthy raw milk with which to meet the widely varying needs of their practice?"

Such denial is very unlikely, he said. "(Nutritional) progress would be much retarded without the aid of Certified milk... with thousands of physicians believing as they do, is it not certain that the profession will always insist that Certified milk be available when needed?"

Certified raw milk was popular from Florida to Hawaii.* There was no question among physicians, especially pediatricians, that raw certified milk was nutritious, safe and therapeutic. Tragically, this knowledge has been forgotten to such an extent that most modern doctors are antagonistic toward raw milk, and they don't even know what "certified" means. What happened?**

The term "raw" should be eliminated from milk grading. It has a connotation in the public mind of a primitive, evil or diseased state as in a raw throat, raw humor, raw sore, or raw meat.

Pasteurized milk should be classified as "Grade B—processed," "Grade B-heated," or "Grade B—pasteurized." Under modern conditions of sanitation, any milk that must be pasteurized to make it safe is inferior milk and should be so labeled. Milk that is homogenized as well as pasteurized should be labeled "Grade C." Only raw certified milk should be labeled "Grade A."

From the American Journal of Public Health, February 1930, "Is it not better public health practice to urge and teach the pasteurization of the lower grades of milk, than to spend time criticizing the non-pasteurization of the highest grade produced?" The American Journal of Public Health, although for pasteurization, clearly recognized that only inferior milk needed pasteurization.

---

* Hawaii had the highest per capita consumption of raw certified milk in the country. Today you could go to jail for selling raw milk in Hawaii. For a state-by-state listing of the legal status of raw milk, see Appendix I.

** The medical school professors, including the veterinary schools, fell for the pasteurization propaganda and dropped the ball. That's what happened.

It probably doesn't surprise you to find that the scientists at the Center for Disease Control (CDC), a federal agency, are just as ignorant as the veterinarians and MD's when it comes to infection and certified milk. From a CDC publication, "An analysis of salmonella cases in the United States in 1979 and 1980 from seventeen states . . . showed that eleven of thirty-two patients had a history of raw milk ingestion.$ Milk from many different dairies was involved. Unlike the tuberculosis and brucellosis, which can be eliminated from dairy herds with precautions, salmonella infections of milking herds continue to occur. Since up to ten percent of healthy cattle may carry salmonella dublin, salmonella contamination of unpasteurized milk can be a persistent problem, *even in dairies that follow the procedures recommended by the American Association of Medical Milk Commissions,* a private organization.

"Present technology cannot produce raw milk (including that listed as certified) that can be assured of being free of pathogens; only with pasteurization is there this assurance. The U.S. Animal Health Association, the National Association of State Public Health Veterinarians, the Conference of State and Territorial Epidemiologists, the American Academy of Pediatrics, and the House of Delegates of the American Veterinarian Association have adopted policy statements that milk for human consumption should be pasteurized. "

This same CDC report[5] stated that there have been two milkborne outbreaks of gastrointestinal disease reported in the United States since 1955. Both were caused bypasteurized milk. Yet in 1981 they have the brass to tell us "only with pasteurization is there assurance" of not getting an intestinal infection from milk.

---

*They undoubtedly also "had a history" of ingesting meat, margarine, eggs, water, and lettuce *which are far more likely to cause salmonella food poisoning than raw milk.* If only one-third (11 of 3 2) of the victims ingested raw milk, what did the other twothirds ingest? Why pick on raw milk?

In 1976, a CDC report showed that the areas with the highest incidence of salmonella food poisoning were Hawaii, New Mexico, District of Columbia, Louisiana, and Massachusetts. *These are all states that do not have raw certified milk.*

Drink raw certified milk for good health, and to hell with the government.

REFERENCES

1. *The History & Analysis of Certified Milk,* Master's, Thesis, P.R. Meyer, University of Georgia, 1979.

2. Annual Convention, Certified Milk Producers Association, Hotel Roosevelt, New York City, February 8, 1938.

3. American Association of Medical Milk Commissions, Proceedings 15th Annual Conference, 1921.

4. Ibid.

5. Family Practice News, September 1, 1981.

Chapter VI

MILKING THE GOOD GUYS

ALTA–DENA

"The Dairy That Cares About Your Health"
(Alta–Dena Motto)

A visit to the Alta-Dena Dairy is an unforgettable experience. It is awesome in size (the largest producer-distributor in the United States). It is automated, computerized, and almost self-sufficient. They make their own plastic containers and grow their own green feed. But in spite of the ultramodern management and gleaming stainless steel computerized equipment in the plant, the offices are in the original buildings and are extremely modest. No thick carpets and expensive furniture. Harold Steuve, the president, shares a cramped office with Boyd Clarke, the assistant manager (his son-in-law). No ostentation here. The offices have that cluttered look of people with plenty to do.

Alta-Dena is definitely a family affair. Not only does practically the whole Steuve clan work for the dairy, but other families have followed their example-two generations of a family may work for the dairy at the same time including brothers, sisters, sons and daughters, aunts and uncles. These family ties have led to a stable and loyal work force. The eight hundred Alta-Dena employees have no union and no need for one. The plant has the air of relaxed efficiency.

There is a paradox at Alta-Dena. Although the plant is a model of American mass production technology, they produce milk just like grandfather used to make-clean, delicious raw milk.

The Steuve brothers, Ed, Harold, and Elmer, set out from their family farm in Frohna, Missouri, to make their fortune in the late 1930's. They all went to work for a dairy in Azusa, California, and by 1945 they had learned enough to operate their own dairy. They purchased a small dairy farm in Monrovia, California and began business in June of 1945 with sixty-one milk cows and two bulls. One month later they started bottling milk and delivering to California households.

As the business grew, the large Steuve clan, consisting of twelve brothers and five sisters, joined the business in California, leaving one brother to manage the farm back in Missouri. Within five years the business had grown so much they needed a new farm. They purchased a much larger operation in Chino, California.

The dairy became officially certified for raw milk in 1953. They grew rapidly following certification. Today the Alta-Dena Dairy totally dominates the certified milk business in California, all of its competitors having given up production because of the cost and difficulty in producing raw certified milk. The dairy milks over eight thousand cows daily and owns eighteen thousand animals. They are the largest producer-distributor in California and the nation. They sell over 20,000 gallons of raw certified milk daily. The lack of disease from this milk is certainly as much proof as anyone could need that raw certified milk is the best and safest to drink.

Alta-Dena has now spread its influence all over the United States, including Alaska and Hawaii. Their products appear in health food stores in practically every state. There are over seventy independent distributors that carry Alta-Dena products in over sixty wholesale routes across the nation. All of their products, which range from

raw certified milk to buttermilk, ice cream, kefir, and yogurt, are entirely free of additives, sugars and dyes.

But it has not been as easy as it may appear, the
company having had relentless persecution from certain
interests, including the health bureaucracy of the state of
California. They have been constantly faced with seizure
of their product, resembling the persecution citizens dis-
tributing Laetrile, DMSO, and other non-government ap-
proved substances have experienced. The attacks often
resemble those conducted on drug pushers. The first as-
sault was in 1965, when a San Diego County health officer summarily banned all raw milk, He said that it
harbored staphlococcus, a virulent organism, which
causes everything from skin infections to penumonia,
septicemia and death. The health officer stated publicly
that he was going to do away with raw milk in the state
of California, if it was the last thing he ever did.

An independent laboratory checked pasteurized and
raw milk samples and found staphlococcus in both milks.
Staph is in everything, including all milk, raw or pasteurized. So what is the rationale behind banning one and not
the other? If all foods containing staph germs were to be
banned, there would be *no fresh food to eat.*

At a hearing of the County Board of Supervisors, the
health officer was asked, "Has anyone become sick from
consuming raw certified milk in San Diego County?" Answer, "No, but it could happen." Although he could not
defend his position on scientific grounds, he refused to
lift the ban, even at the urging of the County Supervisors.

Alta-Dena then instituted a suit against the County
of San Diego. After a three-year battle, the 4th District
Court of Appeals ruled that the health officer had exceeded his authority. Challenging a state health officer,
and winning, was intolerable to the health bureaucrats in
Sacramento. The word went out: Get Alta-Dena Dairy.

In 1967 a resolution by the California Medical Society called for the pasteurization of all milk in Califor-

nia. Fortunately, the legislature was better informed than the doctors and ignored the resolution. Health Officer Askew of San Diego County contacted other counties to combine their forces in an attempt to destroy Alta-Dena's raw certified milk business. Three other counties joined San Diego in banning raw milk. After public opposition grew strong and research proved to them that prohibition was senseless, they rescinded their respective bans, except, of course, for Askew of San Diego County.

Having been rebuffed by the courts, Askew tried a new tactic. He threatened to put up road blocks at the county border to stop the importation of "contraband milk"! The dairy continued to send raw certified milk into San Diego County and the road blocks never materialized.

The Los Angeles County Health Department was next to attack Alta-Dena. This was the Q Fever* caper. In January, 1969, the Los Angeles Times reported, with large headlines, that twenty-nine dairies were selling milk contaminated with Q Fever. The Los Angeles County Health Department had supplied this sensational intelligence to the Times. Alta-Dena raw milk was again banned with the presumption of Q Fever contamination. The dairy defied the order and was taken to court. It was in two courts at once, Los Angeles and San Diego.

The dairy quickly had labels printed describing the raw milk as "pet food, not for human consumption". Mr. Harold Steuve, the president of the dairy and mayor of Monrovia, California, at the time, was arrested for contempt of court. The judge, Los Angeles County health bureaucrats, and the press came out with egg on their faces when it was pointed out by the dairy's experts that Q Fever is caught through inhalation into the lungs and not by drinking milk! The case was dropped.

A county health officer in Southern California, San Bernardino County, snuck a sentence into a bill unrelated

---

*Q Fever is a minor viral disease of little consequence.

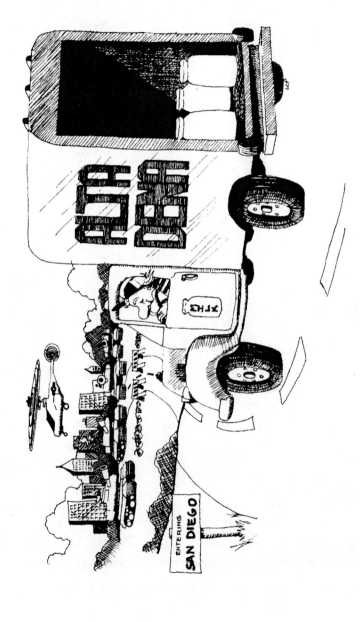

They Vowed to Stop "Contraband Milk" from Entering San Diego.

to raw milk that simply stated, "All milk sold in the county must be pasteurized." This was discovered by accident,* and the enraged county board threw out the bill. When the health officer was interviewed later by Alta-Dena representatives and asked why he attempted such a scurvy trick, they were astounded when he said, "I'm about to retire, and I always wanted to travel around the world."

To show how abysmally ignorant health officials can be, consider the October, 1966, Los Angeles Health Department report of seven Q Fever cases. Six of the seven lived "in or around dairies," they reported, *but none of them drank raw milk.* The mode of spread is *airborne*, they admitted, but "the most practical solution now available" is the universal pasteurization of all milk!

The next attack in this continuing effort to destroy Alta-Dena and unprocessed milk was in 1974, when the Health Department of California, again without any scientific justification whatsoever, condemned the dairy's sale of raw milk because, they claimed, one could contract brucellosis from milk. This attack was absurd, as all Alta-Dena cows are vaccinated against brucellosis. Even though they are vaccinated against brucellosis, the dairy goes the last mile and tests the cows individually.

Again to court. No brucellosis was found in their cows, and Alta-Dena resumed the sale of its unprocessed milk.**

Alta-Dena was next attacked by overly zealous and ignorant health officials because of the possibility, they said, of the dairy's customers getting salmonella food poisoning from unpasteurized milk. The Alta-Dena Dairy and the Medical Milk Commission, which was responsible for the safety of milk, stated that the salmonella would have to be present in the cows' blood to get in the milk, a highly unlikely situation. Not one case of salmo-

---

*Somebody actually read the proposed bill.
**Brucellosis comes from close association with cows and pigs, rarely, if ever, from milk consumption.

nellosis to has been proven to have come from any Alta-Dena milk. Milk samples are tested daily for salmonella. It is highly unlikely that there would be any contamination of milk because of stringent policies required for raw certified milk production.* It is far more likely that one would get salmonella food poisoning from unclean eggs than from raw certified milk.

The attacks by California health officials have been vicious and unrelenting. In one case, a food store operator was forced to pour ninety gallons of raw certified milk down his toilet while the health officer watched! Raw Alta-Dena cheese made in Wisconsin had holes punched in it, and Clorox was poured over the cheese. There was no evidence whatsoever that the milk or the cheese was contaminated. Taking the matter to court, the Alta-Dena Dairy succeeded in winning their case, and the pressure of zealous health officials, at least for the moment, ceased.

A "staff report" from the California Department of Health stated in a widely read publication,[1] "...evidence points to a continuing health hazard to the public consuming Alta-Dena's raw certified milk."

Dr. Ben Werner, a medical epidemiologist with the California Department of Health, said that patients with cancer were being killed by drinking Alta-Dena raw milk.[2] This malicious and irresponsible statement was made in a public magazine read all over California, in spite of the fact that not one person has ever been proven to have even gotten sick from Alta-Dena raw certified milk. The magazine in which he was quoted, New West, is hardly a scientific publication. Using this platform to launch their attack made Werner and his colleague, Dr. C.L. Humphrey, look more like propagandists than scientists. But they found a way around that. Their highly misleading and inaccurate material was published in England,

---

* Finding salmonella in feces does not mean that it will be in the milk.

where checking of the facts would be more difficult, but where they could trade on their positions as officials of the California Department of Health. The British Medical Journal would have no reason to suspect that Werner and Humphrey were merely on a vendetta to destroy the Alta-Dena Dairy, using propaganda rather than scientific fact.

The British article was a beaut, again claiming that Alta-Dena raw certified milk had killed helpless cancer patients due to salmonella.*

After having slipped this article through a foreign publication that would be relatively immune from lawsuits, American medical publications could then quote it as *scientific fact*. The Journal of Public Health Policy, a journal for medical bureaucrats, quoted the article extensively. Others have followed suit leaving Alta-Dena with an image of malfeasance.

A young inspector for the California Department of Food and Agriculture told a lurid tale to the press of seeing sores on animals, "so big I could put both feet in them and still have room to turn around." Although the statement is ridiculous on its face, no cow with a sore *two feet in diameter* could escape notice in even the worst dairy and certainly not in the dairy chosen by the United States Department of State as the *official showcase dairy for foreign visitors.***

These attacks caused an almost unbelievable reaction from the people of California. By August of 1978, the governor's office had received over seventeen thousand letters, telegrams, and phone calls in defense of Alta-Dena.

---

* Most cancer patients die from some sort of terminal infection. It may be salmonella, stapMococcus, Torula Histolytica (a fungus) or any other of dozens of pathogens. This is often aided and abetted by cancer doctors giving powerful chemical compounds that destroy the patients'resistance. Some call this chemo-euthanasia. Even raw certified milk can't protect the patient from that.

** Everyone loves Alta-Dena but the California bureaucrats.

No one knows how many letters have been received by now, but it is well over fifty thousand.*

There was a furious legislative battle in 1978. The Steuve brothers were attempting to get legislation passed that would call off the bureaucratic dogs of war. It would appear from the record that state health officials went so far as to falsify bacterial reports in an attempt to discredit the dairy at the time this legislation was being considered.[3]

When the state laboratory claimed the milk was positive (contaminated), a laboratory testing for the Los Angeles County Milk Commission and a laboratory which does considerable testing for the state retested their samples, and again the milk proved to be negative. There can only be two possible explanations for the discrepancy between the laboratories: the state deliberately falsified its testing results, or their methods are so sloppy that the milk samples were contaminated during the testing procedures.

Inflammatory headlines:

"Raw Milk Warning" - San Rafael Independent Journal, June 10, 1978.

"Some Raw Milk Found to be Contaminated" - Star Free Press, Ventura, California, June 11, 1978.

"New Warning on Alta-Dena Raw Milk Told" - Press Telegram, Long Beach, California, June 10, 1980.

"Contaminated Milk Ordered Off Shelves" - Sacramento Union, June 15, 1978.

There were radio announcements warning people, "not to drink raw milk from Alta-Dena Dairy."

---

*Californians believe in God, country - and Alta-Dena raw certified milk.

For those who think government agencies are above conspiring against a private company, explain this. The state laboratory made its "discovery" that a batch of Alta-Dena raw certified milk was contaminated on June 4, 1978. The Senate bill that would prevent the state health department from harassing the Alta-Dena Dairy was to be considered the following week. Instead of immediately releasing their alarming findings that people were going to get sick from salmonella food poisoning and that a possible epidemic was in the offing from "contaminated" raw milk, the press was not notified until the evening of June 9, just before the hearing! If the state laboratory had been correct in their findings, in the intervening five days *ten thousand or more* people could have been sick from salmonella food poisoning.

In December, the controversy started all over again:

"State Issues Warning about Alta-Dena Milk" - Argus, Fremont, California, December 9, 1978.

"Dairy's Raw Milk Again Under Fire" - Hemet News, Hemet, California, December 9, 1978.

"Poisoned Milk Recalled" - Richmond Post, Oakland, California, December 15, 1978.

In February, 1979, the attacks, like a broken record, started all over again:

"Tainted Milk Ordered Off Market Shelves" - San Gabriel Valley Tribune, Covina, California, February 10, 1979.

Again, the allegations were completely false.

Things really got rough after Alta-Dena sued the state for $80,000,000 in damages. The state counterattacked. Assemblyman William Dannemyer, who had

been the Alta-Dena attorney, began receiving some direct
hits. His opponent for a Congressional seat, Bill Farris,
announced to the press that the FBI had visited him concerning Dannemyer's possible "dealings with lobbyists"
for Alta-Dena Dairy.* No investigation ever took place.

A letter to the editor of the Fullerton Tribune,
Fullerton, California, said this about the Bill Farris attack,
"...Farris... seems to make a habit of suing his political
opponents on charges that can't hold up in court...
Dannemyer ...has continued to speak on the issue clearly
without sinking to Farris' mud-slinging level."

Dannemyer was elected to the United States House
of Representatives where he continues to serve with dis-
tinction. His only regret: You can't get raw milk in Washington.

After observing the Los Angeles County Certified
Milk Commission in action, I can only conclude that the
Commission is useless. Its members are sincere men who
believe they are serving the high standards set by the
Methods and Standards of the Milk Commission. But when
the six commission members have to listen to the harangues
of the health department and spend all of their commission
time investigating the harassment of the only dairy in the
state that has a vested interest in producing the cleanest
milk possible, it becomes an exercise in futility.

There are twenty dairies in California selling
uncertified raw milk. This milk, in some cases, is processed under highly questionable conditions. *None of these
dairies meet the standards of certified milk as does the Alta-
Dena Dairy, and they are not inspected by the Milk Commission.* The commission exists solely for the purpose of
inspecting the two dairies that are interested in producing milk under this high standard. A member of the Milk

---

*Now why would the FBI visit a political opponent with no
connection whatsoever to the milk industry?

Commission admitted to me privately, "The whole thing is crazy. It's a complete waste of time."*

The State Health Department is responsible for inspecting other than certified dairies. The average dairy may get inspected ten times a year, if that.

It should be noted that even raw milk produced under less than ideal circumstances, that is, not under certified standards, seldom causes disease. Although their record is not as good as that of Alta-Dena (which is, for all intents and purposes, perfect), they have been responsible for very little infectious disease. Most outbreaks have been caused by foods other than milk. This illustrates the fact that raw milk, if produced with just a modicum of cleanliness, is safe because of built-in safeguards that have not been destroyed by heating. These built-in safeguards are aided by modern refrigeration. But to be on the safe side,** don't drink raw milk unless it is certified.

Conclusion: Require *all milk* to be certified to retain a safe and nutritious product for everyone.

With all the adverse publicity, someone was bound to sue the dairy eventually. It is remarkable that, in spite of overt and covert encouragement by public health officials, only one case has come to court.

Mary Smith (fictitious name) sued Alta-Dena Certified Dairy for damages, alleging pain and suffering due to contracting food poisoning from Alta-Dena raw certified milk. The bacteria isolated by the county and the California Public Health Department from Smith was salmonella montevideo. She blamed her condition on Alta-Dena raw certified milk even though she had had repeated episodes of diarrheal disease for *over a year* prior to the consumption of the raw milk; her doctors refused to testify that raw milk was responsible; and *salmonella montevideo doesn't even occur in milk*, raw or otherwise.

---

* No, I can't tell you his name. He needs to stay on the Milk Commission.

** And protect me from lawsuits.

Such is the power of the press. The case was laughed out of court.

A fourteen-year-old boy contracted salmonella gastroenteritis. He could never remember drinking raw milk, although the family members, (who did *not* get sick), did drink Alta-Dena raw certified milk. As it turned out, the young man and his friend had been playing a little game of spitting *toilet bowl water* at each other. That's probably as good a method as any of *guaranteeing* a good case of salmonella gastroenteritis. The health department labeled it as an "Alta-Dena associated case"!

I have in my files many more equally preposterous cases. Alta-Dena has initiated an $80,000,000 suit against the state for harassment. And, as this book was being written, the California Health Department renewed the attack. A report of February, 1981, said:

> "Salmonellae have been recovered forty-five times since 1977 from California-produced raw milk that was distributed. All of the isolates were made from Alta-Dena's raw certified milk, taken both before and after bottling. Since Alta-Dena produces about ninety percent of raw milk sold in California, that dairy will more than likely be involved... when raw milk is found to be contaminated, or when raw milk is found to be associated with human illness.
>
> Previously, Alta-Dena had been identified in an investigation of one hundred-thirteen human cases of Salmonella Dublin infection that occurred statewid... of those cases...thirty-one percent used Alta-Dena raw certified milk."

As these are sophisticated men of science, it is hard to believe that this report, entirely false, was not deliberate and malicious. If not deliberate, then the Great Black Hole of Ignorance among medical scientists, at least in California, is indeed stupefying.*

---

* In a survey of California legislators, the Department of Health was rated the worst in the state government. It was described as "inefficient, incompetent, and unresponsive." As you might expect, they get the most money—over four billion dollars a year.

In 1982 and 1983 the battle shifted to Nevada. State inspectors seized some Alta-Dena milk from a health food store and claimed that it contained salmonella. The milk was 21 days old.*

The California State Health Department, not one to miss an opportunity, went for the Alta-Dena jugular. In spite of the fact that the Food and Drug Administration, after three days of intensive investigation, found nothing of importance at the Alta-Dena lab; in spite of a clean bill of health on the milk (although it was 21 days old) from four different labs, *including two of their own state and county labs*, the health department issued warnings to the people of California not to drink Alta-Dena raw milk or even give it to their pets!

When the state issues these propaganda attacks against Alta-Dena, consumers call the dairy in a panic. Paul Virgin, publicity director, tells them, "If you are worried about the milk, bring it in. We'll give you your money back, and I'll drink the milk."**

Perhaps the most bizarre accusation against the dairy concerned a miscarriage. A 300-pound diabetic woman refused to heed the warnings of doctors. Two doctors would not take her case because of her irresponsibility. A midwife eventually delivered twins, decayed and stillborn and the whole mess was blamed on Alta-Dena raw milk!

Maybe you think California Health Department bureaucrats are a special breed, more vicious and stupid than most. Let's move over to Georgia and check out their health bureaucrats.

It's a special situation in Georgia because they have the Feds in the Center for Disease Control as well as their own homegrown variety of bureaucrat.

---

* Alta-Dena, like any other food company, can't protect the consumer from irresponsible merchants. They shouldn't sell spoiled milk any more than spoiled meat.

** Sometimes he drinks the condemned milk on television.

ROSEBUD AND MATHIS DAIRY

The name Mathis is as familiar to Atlantans as Margaret Mitchell. Even people who don't buy Mathis milk, including their competitors, will tell you that Mathis Certified Dairy is a quality operation. The dairy mascot, "Rosebud," is known to every school child in the surrounding counties. An average of two hundred fifty people a day visit the dairy on tours, and most of the children take a hand at milking "Rosebud."

Raw milk sells well in Atlanta because the people trust Mathis. But, as with Alta-Dena, it hasn't been easy. The dairy was founded in 1917. Mr. Mathis, called "Mr. Lloyd" by just about everybody, is now 85 years old. His son Jack runs the dairy and has been the inspiration for the raw milk crusade in the southeastern United States. Without Mathis and Alta-Dena fighting this lonely battle at opposite ends of the country, there would be absolutely no nutritious milk available in this country.

In the 50's, a law was passed in Georgia that allowed the sale of raw certified milk only by prescription of an M.D. This was a cumbersome, unworkable law that made it extremely difficult for consumers to obtain raw milk. That, of course, was the intent of the law.

Frustrated by this unfair and discriminatory law, Jack Mathis, President of Mathis Certified Dairy in Decatur, Georgia, told the Commissioner of Agriculture that he was going to sell raw certified milk to anyone who wanted it *with or without* a prescription. This got everyone's attention, and a bill was soon introduced to take the restrictions off the sale of raw certified milk in Georgia.

All hell broke loose. Not since the War Between the States* had there been such turmoil and show of emotion in the Georgia legislature. For forty days and forty nights the debate raged on. The state health department, the Univer-

---

*Called the "Civil War" up North.

sity of Georgia, all of the dairy organizations, the Medical Association of Georgia, and even the Parent/Teachers Association worked themselves up into an emotional lather. You would have thought, watching this circus, that Mathis Dairy was trying to sell raw sewage rather than raw milk. In the minds of many of these hysterical, wellmeaning, but uninformed people, one was as bad as the other.

Members of the Parent/Teacher Association picketed the capitol building carrying signs imploring the legislature to "Save Pasteurized Milk for our Children." Pasteurized milk, of course, wasn't even the issue. One member of the legislature said that passage of the bill allowing the unrestricted sale of raw certified milk would be "going back to the dark ages."

Dairy President Jack Mathis asked a learned professor during the heated debate, "Don't you think people should be allowed to choose what they eat?" He replied, "No! It's time we *legislate* what people eat."*

Organized dairy interests put out a "fact sheet" to convince legislators that they should vote against this bill to legalize the sale of raw certified milk. The fact sheet said that "no responsible dairy organization" in the state of Georgia supported the bill.** This included the Georgia Dairy Association, the Georgia Farm Bureau, and the Georgia Association of Dairy Cooperatives. The fact sheet also pointed out that "all government health agencies" and state school authorities were opposed to the bill.

---

* Professors, like government bureaucrats, are prone to think that they know what's best for you. They may have to force you to drink pasteurized, homogenized milk, but it's for your own good.
** What they *should* have said was that none of the dairy organizations with a vested interest in producing cheap, cleanedup, dirty milk supported the bill.

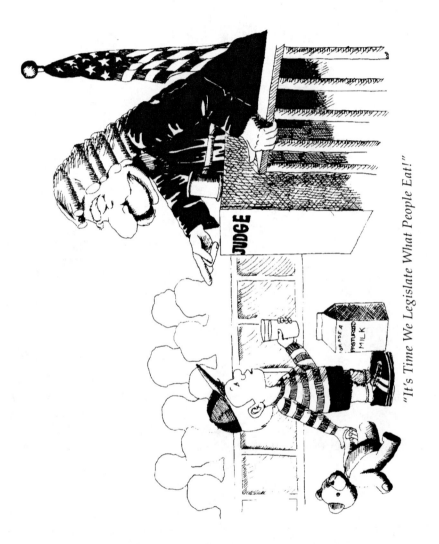

"It's Time We Legislate What People Eat!"

The only groups supporting the bill, the fact sheet said, were "food faddists" and one little local dairy that "stands to gain commercially."*

It was Mathis Certified Dairy against the world, or so it seemed. But there was one other group that backed the Mathis determination to produce clean milk. It was the people of Georgia. The bill passed the House by an overwhelming majority.

The pasteurization fanatics didn't fold. The bill passed the Senate and then went back to the House for final approval. Clever, delaying tactics resulted in the bill dying because of adjournment of the Georgia legislature. The will of the people had been thwarted—or so it seemed.

But they underestimated the courage and determination of Jack Mathis. He called the Secretary of Agriculture and informed him that, since the people of Georgia had expressed their will, he would not let legislative double-dealing stop the flow of clean milk to his customers.

A legislative hearing was set. At the hearing, one of the Department of Agriculture attorneys took young Mathis aside and whispered in his ear, "If my mama knew I was down here opposing Rosebud, she would *kill* me. I was raised on your milk!"

Mathis lost. The case was sent to Superior Court for a decision. The Superior Court reversed the decision of the Department of Agriculture and Mathis Dairy continued to serve the people of Georgia with clean, unadulterated milk.

As we found out in California, bureaucrats will never forgive you for beating them in court.** Mathis received

---

* Producing clean raw milk is an expensive process. Most people don't understand that clean certified milk is worth the difference in price. Mathis would be better off financially just to forget about raw certified milk.

** They think the courts are *theirs* to be used to carry out *their* will.

national publicity when he went to Iowa to defend a dairyman who was selling raw milk. When he got home, he found *seven physicians* at the dairy, sent by the Center for Disease Control, to inspect the dairy herd. The State of Georgia hadn't been able to send Rosebud to the slaughterhouse, so the Feds took over.

"It looked like germ warfare had set in," Mathis said. They checked *every cow* once, twice, and then a third time. After a long delay, the CDC admitted that their inspectors had found nothing.*

While this "inspection" was going on, the CDC was attacking on another flank. The experts at CDC decided to make an issue of campylobacter, a mild gastrointestinal disease that causes diarrhea. They conducted a survey of households in an attempt to link campylobacter infections to Mathis raw certified milk. They found no correlation between infection and Mathis milk, but they were able to turn their "survey" into a propaganda campaign against the dairy anyway.

A typical case was the housewife who called to cancel her milk order. The Center for Disease Control agents had confused and frightened her. Her ten-month-old baby had diarrhea. The agents told her that the infection was campylobacter caused by Mathis raw milk.

"I don't understand how they came to that conclusion," she told Mr. Mathis. "I told them, 'Look, my husband is the big milk drinker, and he didn't get sick. My ten-month-old *doesn't drink the milk*, but he's the one who got sick. Do you think I'm a moron?' For some reason, they're really out to get you, Mr. Mathis."

A man called to cancel his raw milk order. The CDC told him that his pregnant wife's campylobacter infection was caused by Mathis raw certified milk. "And not only that," he exclaimed, "she gave it to my two dogs!"**

---

* Very few dairies could withstand such a rigorous inspection. A certified dairy will pass every time.

** How did she do that?

Where does this unpronounceable campylobacter germ come from? It comes primarily from poultry, especially chicken and turkey, *and the water* that comes out of your kitchen faucet.*

The CDC remains unconcerned about these major sources of the infection.** They look even more ridiculous (and conspiratorial) when it is realized that *campylobacter has neuer been recovered from raw milk*. The reason for this is simple, and the CDC knows it: raw milk contains lactoperoxidase which inactivates campylobacter.[6]

A high official asked Jack Mathis: "Why don't you just sell out and retire rich? Why fight it?"

"I will continue to sell clean milk to the people of Georgia," he replied. "When I am no longer allowed to sell unadulterated milk, I will close the dairy."

Mathis and Alta-I)ena set an example for the rest of the country, but they need your help. Form a group to influence your state legislators. Call it MAMA—Mothers Against Milk Adulteration.*** Buy and distribute this book.**** Ask your dairy why it doesn't produce milk clean enough not to need heating. If Mathis and Alta-Dena can do it, why can't they?

---

* Flying poultry, known as birds, poop into tho water supply.

** 22% of chicken samples from retail stores have been found to be contaminated with campylobacter; 94% of turkey.[5]

*** Maybe you can think of a better name.

**** I have to make a living too.

REFERENCES

1. New West, August 14, 1978.

2. Ibid.

3. Los Angeles Herald Examiner, June 15, 1978.

4. Santa Ana Register, June 11, 1978.

5. Luechtefeld, J. Chem. Microbiol., 13:266-268.

6. Doyle & Roman, Appl. Environ. Microbiol., 44:1154-1158.

Chapter VII

UDDER MENACE—
HOMOGENIZATION OF MILK

You've got to learn two new words. They are "plasmalogen" and "XO".*

Current dogma says that saturated fat, especially animal fat, and cholesterol are the culprits in atherosclerosis. A look at eating patterns over the past eighty years will reveal how unlikely it is that animal fat and cholesterol are the causes of hardening of the arteries. We discuss this in detail in Chapter XII. A review of food patterns shows that animal fat consumption has not changed materially since 1900. If animal fat consumption is the cause of atherosclerosis, then why was it an uncommon disease before the mid-20th century?

How does one explain the Masai tribe of East Africa? The Masai are cattle herders. Their diet is nothing but meat, milk, and blood. That's as high a fat and cholesterol diet as you can get. Yet atherosclerosis is practically unknown among the Masai tribesmen.

The fat-cholesterol school of atherogenesis** had an answer to this paradox. The Masai have an incredibly high level of physical activity. They walk as much as sixty miles a day. The exercise, they said, was the reason the Masai had low blood cholesterol levels and little hardening of the arteries.

---

* Keep hold of these words, because they're the key to understanding why homogenized milk can kill you. XO stands for xanthine oxidase, an enzyme.
** Atherogenesis: causing hardening of the arteries.

This sounded pretty good until another group of scientists pointed to the natives of East Finland. These lumberjack types expend more energy chopping wood than the Masai do walking sixty miles a day. Yet, they have the highest death rate in the world from atherosclerotic heart disease.

The reason the lumberjacks had such a high incidence of heart disease, the animal fat theorists said, was because of the high animal fat and cholesterol content of their diet. And they proved it, they claimed, by cutting down the animal fat level of the East Finnish population. There was a dramatic decrease in the degree of atherosclerotic heart disease with a switch to vegetable fat.

Conclusive proof—right?*

While they were altering the diet, the team of researchers also conducted an intensive (and successful) anti-smoking campaign. The lumberjacks were very heavy smokers. *The reduction in smoking was clearly the major factor, and probably the only factor, leading to a decrease in heart attacks.* The decrease in smoking was a strong enough factor to overcome the unwise reduction in consumption of animal fat and increase in vegetable fat.

What about primitive Eskimos? They eat *blubber*. But they have little atherosclerotic heart disease.**

Acting on faulty statistics or at least statistics that in themselves had no significance, the spokesmen for organized medicine recommended that Americans make changes in their diet by reducing the consumption of saturated animal fat and cholesterol. The American people took their advice halfway. They did not decrease animal fat consumption significantly, but they greatly increased their consumption of vegetable fats and the situation got worse.

---

* Wrong.

** On a trip to the Arctic Circle, I tried some blubber. I guess they eat it because they have to.

If saturated animal fat consumption hasn't changed, what has changed that would cause an increase in atherosclerosis? You will find out what vegetable fat does to your arteries in the Margarine chapter, but Dr. Kurt A. Oster says that the homogenization of milk is another major cause of atherosclerosis.

In the homogenization process, the fat particles of the cream are broken up. This is done by straining the fat through tiny pores under great pressure. The resulting fat particles are so small (one-millionth of a meter) that they stay in suspension. So the cream is evenly distributed throughout the milk. Most Americans under the age of forty have never seen milk in its natural state with a cream layer. They have been so programmed to drinking milk with an even texture that the sight of cream floating on milk is usually met with revulsion. It looks yacky to the modern eye.

Oster, Zikakis, and other investigators discovered that the substance plasmalogen* was depleted in the areas of the heart where a blockage had taken place. The walls of the arteries not affected by the atherosclerotic process contained the normal amount of plasmalogen. Where the arteries were hardened, XO had replaced the plasmalogen.

So they began to look around for the possible dietary source of the XO. Dairy products, they discovered, are the only source of this lethal enzyme.** But milk and milk products have been a source of food for centuries. Heart disease is a disease of modern times. At least it wasn't common until the 20th century. What had happened to cause XO to be absorbed into the bloodstream, attack plasmalogen, and then deposit on the arteries? What significant changes had taken place in milk processing?

The first big change was pasteurization which has contributed greatly to the degenerative disease epidemics, including atherosclerosis. The other radical change was homogenization.

---

* Did you remember it?
** Human milk contains no XO.

XO, Oster discovered, was attached to the fat globules of milk. Normal fat globules are too big to go through the gut wall and into the blood stream. But after homogenization, they pass through easily. They increase in number some one-hundred times and with them goes the deadly XO.

Critics said that absorption of XO from the intestine was impossible because it was such a large molecule. The XO must be "endogenous," that is, from the human liver. As with many "impossible" things in science, XO absorption from the intestine was only impossible to those who wished they had discovered it first. Gregoriadis and Weissmant proved that these large molecules are indeed absorbed and thereby they opened new avenues of thought and research in medicine.*

But the critics still were not silenced. Okay, they said, maybe it *could* be absorbed, but it won't be because that large a molecule (XO) can't survive the digestive process in the stomach and small intestine, "Not possible." Gregoriadis and Zikakis again proved them wrong.[2] They proved that some remarkable little armored cars called "liposomes"** do indeed protect XO from digestive enzymes and carry them into the blood stream.

The milk industry says don't worry, pasteurization kills the XO. It does kill some of it.*** But at the 170° F pasteurization temperatures, 40% of the XO is left in the active state.

We've got another problem. You know that Vitamin D the milk producers have so kindly added to your milk? In the first place, it isn't a vitamin. It's a hormone like cortisone. Second, *it's helping XO harden your arteries.*

---

* If big *bad* molecules, like XO, could be absorbed through the gut, then so could big *good* molecules, like antibodies. See Chapter XI.

** You don't have to remember that.

*** Along with all the good enzymes you need for good health.

Doctors Ross and Oster[3] have discovered that D_3, the one they add to pasteurized milk and other processed foods, activates XO. In the presence of testosterone, the male sex hormone, it activates XO even more. So a male, drinking pasteurized, homogenized, Vitamin D, "Grade A" milk is really asking for it.

Dr. Oster discovered that the B vitamin, folic acid, is protective against the destructive effects of XO. You shouldn't drink pasteurized, Grade A, etc., etc., under any circumstances, but if you insist upon drinking it, take a folic acid supplement with B12.*

A Univeristy of California group did a study on XO and reported that Oster was wrong. They said XO was absorbed in only infinitesimal amounts. Their experiments were vague and irrelevant. They made no attempt to actually repeat Oster's experiments which is the way to prove or disprove a piece of research. The California report, which merely served to confuse the issue, was funded by big cash from the homogenization gang—the National Dairy Council.**

Oster's work has since been largely confirmed at the University of Delaware. The American Heart Association continues to look the other way and pursue dangerous chemicals as a treatment for atherosclerosis. Most of the American Heart Association's bills are paid by drug company advertising, and, "If industry pays the tab..."

There are other reasons for not homogenizing milk. One of them is "taint". That's not just a southern colloqui–alism for ain't. In the dairy industry it refers to a

---

* You will then have a false sense of security and can enjoy the calcium dystrophy syndrome, colitis, and bad teeth.

** That's known as udder politics or, as researchers from this same university put it: "Money can influence –or dictate– what research gets done. If industry pays the tab, they've got a right to call the tune."[5]

deterioration of the milk fat leading to off-flavors vari-
ously described as a "cardboard," "oily," or "tallowy"
taste. The more of the surface of the fat that is exposed to
oxidation, the more the taint. Homogenization greatly increases the amount of fat surface. There are friendly bacteria in milk that aid in preventing oxidation of the fat.
The enzyme catalase also helps by inactivating oxygen.
But both of them, the friendly bacteria and the catalase,
went up the flue when the milk was pasteurized. No
wonder milk doesn't taste like the good old days, and
consumption continues to decline.

As we were about to button up this book, an epidemic
of cholesterol phobia again gripped the nation. The Journal
of the American Medical Association reported work done by
the National Heart, Lung and Blood Institute* that proved
cholesterol is Public Enemy Number One.

Tom Valentine, reporting in the weekly newspaper
Spotlight, called it "Commercial Science"—science directed toward improving marketability. "The stakes are
high," he said, "the vegetable oil industry rides the crest
of the anti-cholesterol wave."

The Reader's Digest entered the anti-cholesterol war
in their June, 1984 edition. This government report, they
said, "put an end to wishful thinking." Dietary cholesterol is the killer.**

Dr. Oster wrote a blistering and well-reasoned challenge to the AMA report. The Journal of the American
Medical Association refused to *prin tit*. Butthe newspaper
Spotlight has a penchant for puncturing pompous and
pusillanimous publications. They gave it good coverage
in the August 27, 1984 issue.

The AMA report was naive at best. Using a potent
and dangerous drug, cholestyramine, the Journal of the

---

* Be suspicious of any group whose title starts out with "National". You
know what happens when bureaucrats try to help you.

** Remember what the Reader's Digest told you about raw milk? See
Chapter IV.

American Medical Association reported that lowering the serum cholesterol reduced the number of heart attacks in the treated group as compared with "control" patients that didn't receive the drug. Oster pointed out that the total mortality was reduced by *0.1 percent.* You don't need a degree in statistics to realize that one in a thousand improvement is meaningless.

What *was* significant was the 175% increase in deaths due to violence and accidents in the drug-treated group.*

This was supposed to have been a "double blind" study.* But most of the patients on the drug were *throwing* up, so they knew they were on the drug and so did their doctor.***

I'll tell you something that might give you a coronary. This "scientific" study costs you, the taxpayer, 150 million dollars. This report was also an insult to Dr. Oster's fine research. Xanthene oxidase from the homogenization of milk as a major factor in atherosclerosis was not even mentioned.

Here are the reasons for not drinking homogenized milk.

1) An increased susceptibility to spoilage because of fat surface exposure.
2) XO absorption into your bloodstream with consequent hardening of the arteries.
3) Tainting.
4) Increased fat absorption beyond what nature intended with unknown effect.

Here are the reasons for drinking homogenized milk:

1) You can't get anything but homogenized milk and, besides...

---

* Cholestyramine drives some people wacky.

** Neither patient nor doctor is supposed to know whether the patient is taking a placebo or the drug.

*** Powerful drugs always have side effects. That's why double blind studies are usually worthless.

2) The Federal Trade Commission says that homogenization is harmless, and homogenized milk is a "natural product."
3) You don't believe what I have told you about homogenized milk and, anyway...
4) You like playing Russian roulette with your health.

REFERENCES

1. Weissman, Ann. New York Academy Science, 308,235, 1978.

2. Zikakis, et al, J. Dairy Science, 60, 533, 1977.

3. Personal telephone interview with Dr. Donald J. Ross, Fairfield University, January, 1982.

4. Oster, A.J.C.R., Volume II, #1, April, 1971.

5. Nutrition Today, November/December, 1981, pp. 29.

6. The Spotlight, Aug. 27, 1984.

Chapter VIII

UDDER FOLLY

Pasteurized, homogenized milk is bad enough, but wait until you hear about the milk substitutes.

You may now purchase, from your neighborhood grocer, pasteurized, homogenized dipotassium and calcium phosphate, with hydrogenated vegetable fat, sodium caseinate, sugar (of course), artificial flavoring (of course), guar gum, "NATURAL color,"* carrageenan, salt, and all blended with that wonderful food, sodium silicoaluminate.** This chemical concoction looks like milk and tastes somewhat like milk. But there the resemblance ends.

One manufacturer of pseudo milk guarantees the distributor that there are no more than 20,000 bacteria per cubic centimeter. That's twice the allowable bacteria count of raw certified milk. We had a sample of one of these industrial wonders tested by the Georgia Department of Agriculture. They found *110,000* bacteria per cubic centimeter! Bugs just love to grow in powdered milk and milk substitutes.

The fat used in most of these ersatz milk preparations is coconut oil. They use coconut oil because it is

---

* The company capitalized the word"NATURAL."They're proud of that.
** To those of you who are not chemistry professors, that is also known as sand.

cheap. That's also why they use it in soap.* But I'll bet you haven't eaten soap since you were a kid and your mother caught you saying "s--t". At least you knew what you were eating.** They also use coconut oil in some baby formulas. Gets the kids off to a good start. See Chapter IX.

One of the biggest get-rich schemes since the Florida land boom and the Dutch tulip craze is the high-powered promotion now going on for these milk substitutes made from the waste product of cheese production called whey.

Business has been so phenomenal that the companies have gone into night shifts according to one promoter. Automated equipment has been installed that will enable them to produce *7500* pounds a minute. Even America's super cows look like lactating mice by comparison. The profits? The last time we checked, it was well over a million dollars a day. As greed fever abates, this figure will undoubtedly fall. There are only so many suckers to go around.

How do they do it? It's similar to the old pyramid game, but now called multi-level selling: buy one, sell one, get them to sell one, etc. It works whether you are selling soap or phony milk.***

The dairymen used to throw the whey down the drain, but it clogged the sewers. They tried fermenting it for methane gas production. That was unsuccessful. Feeding it to the pigs seemed a good idea, but even the pigs didn't like it, so they used it for fertilizer. It's known as "the whey disposal problem."[1]

The general rule seems to be, "When all else fails, feed it to humans." So a Salt Lake City outfit took whey

---

* It makes great soap. Safeguard, Lifebuoy, and Dove are all made from coconut oil.

** It's a wise man who knows his fodder.

*** It's the American way. I just don't think phony milk is good for you or your family.

residue, threw in some sugar, coconut oil, a bunch of GRAS chemicals* and five synthetic vitamins, and presto—a product that is "33% to 42% more nutritious than milk"!

Pigs and people wouldn't eat whey because it tastes awful. But junk food promoters have proven that the American people will eat anything if you put enough sugar and artificial flavoring in it and call it "natural" and "nutritious." The stuff is selling like ten-cent gasoline. People won't drink gasoline,** but beleaguered by high prices, the American people are looking for cheap food substitutes. The food industry has found the way, although the eventual cost in bad health will be heavy indeed.

We used to be concerned about atherosclerosis in young adults. Korean War autopsy studies revealed advanced atherosclerosis in eighteen year olds. But we now see atherosclerosis in *childhood*! Counterfeit milk is not the sole cause, or probably a major cause (yet) for the physical degeneration that we are witnessing. But it can be added to bogus butter, chemical ice cream, cola drinks and other industrial solvents, swimming pool grade drinking water, packaged sugar bombs called power-packed breakfast foods and fast food restaurants serving quickie foods composed primarily of embalmed meat, fish or chicken fried in coconut oil.

Back in the old days, skim milk was called "Blue John" because of its bluish tint. Skim and low-fat milk would not have reached their present state of popularity, in spite of doctors recommending it, without considerable manipulation to improve the taste. Skim and low-fat milk simply don't have the rich flavor and consistency of

---

* GRAS stands for "GenerallyRegardedAs Safe."Doesn't that make you feel secure? Red Dye #2 was a GRAS chemical until they found it causes cancer in laboratory animals. It is no longer GRAS since they found it will put you under the grass.

** Maybe they would ff you added enough sugar and GRAS chemicals.

whole milk. But the food technologists could make saw-
dust taste good if someone created a market for it.* To
give the Blue John "body, texture, and mouth-feel," a
technical bulletin says,[2] you add Crest Lac #300. This
additive is a superheated dry milk. The protein is "dena-
tured"** and "modified." The process is patented, so they
won't tell you what happens when they "modify" it.***
Feed it to a baby calf, and he'll die.

Why do they use this stuff instead of regular dry
milk? You guessed it. It's cheaper. Look at the label on
your skim milk bottle, "Grade A pasteurized skimmed
milk with high heat to increase absorption— 'Superheated' Grade A nonfat milk solids added." Now you
know what that means —junk food.

"Filled" milk was one of the first adulterations of natural milk. Fifty years ago Congress enacted legislation prohibiting the interstate transportation of this doctored
product made from skim milk and vegetable oil.

One Charles Hauser, a dairy farmer from Illinois
who was in the filled milk business, spent a fortune
fighting the Filled Milk Act and went to jail rather than
give in.**** With the present fat and cholesterol obsession of scientists, filled milk has enjoyed a revival, and
Hauser would appear to have been ahead of his time. In
1973 the federal courts declared the Filled Milk Act unconstitutional. The Food and Drug Administration declared that filled milk was a safe and nutritious
food.*****

---

* As a matter of fact they have. They put it in some brands of bread
and call it "fibre."

** That's a very descriptive word. It means the protein is no longer as
nature intended. The nature has been taken out.

*** After you denature or kill something, you have to embalm it, right?

**** Being dedicated to a cause doesn't necessarily make you right.

*****That should make you suspicious.

Because of the relentless propaganda of the cholesterolfat school of nutrition and the unceasing efforts of the ersatz milk manufacturers, consumption of unadulterated milk, that is raw milk, is practically nonexistent except in Georgia and California. Consumption of pasteurized, homogenized milk is also declining because of the cholesterol propaganda. While we do not lament the decline in pasteurized, homogenized milk consumption, *it is a nutritional disaster that fresh raw milk is being thrown out along with the bad milk,* and "filled milk" is gaining in popularity. It is guilt by association. Not enough people understand the problem. So milk substitutes have taken 30% of the dairy market.

The word got around that I was going to zap ersatz milk in this book. Then one day, Wham! The president of Meadow Fresh, the largest of the imitation milk producers, landed in my office.

President Roy Brog created Meadow Fresh.* He is not without credentials, having obtained his master's degree in dairy science from Utah State University.** He sincerely believes in his product. He said that people have come to him with tears in their eyes to thank him for creating Meadow Fresh. He is a man with a mission.

When asked how much money the company was making, he declined to say.*** However, he did reveal that the company has one hundred thousand distributors and produces 400,000 gallons of product every day. The production, he said, will soon double. Not bad for a company that is only a few years old.

---

* What a misnomer. It doesn't come from a meadow, but a laboratory and it sure as hell isn't fresh.

** I checked him out.

*** I knew it was none of my business, but I just wondered.

Meadow Fresh claims to have improved on Mother Nature's natural product:

— 40% more nutritious than milk.

— A suitable substitute for milk for babies over 12 months of age.

— Costs less than milk. — Low in fat.

— Suitable for those with allergies to milk.

A review by the Utah Trade Commission and the Utah State Department of Agriculture resulted in an order by the State of Utah to Meadow Fresh Farms to modify some of its claims. An agreement, dated July 29, 1981, was filed stating that Meadow Fresh will change its labels, promotional materials and marketing information so as not to mislead the consuming public in the following areas:

• Meadow Fresh products will not be represented for use in infant formulas.

• Meadow Fresh products will not be represented as containing no cholesterol.

• Meadow Fresh products will not be represented as being equal to, nutritionally superior to, or directly comparable with cow's or human milk.

• Meadow Fresh products will not be represented as being suitable for consumption by persons who are allergic to milk without any adverse reactions.

• Meadow Fresh products will not be represented as being curative for various diseases and illnesses.

Alaska went further. They hit Meadow Fresh with a fine. Meadow Fresh admitted to charges brought against them by the Alaska attorney general[3] that they had made false or misleading claims about the cholesterol and calorie content of Meadow Fresh, government "approval" of their product and its nutritional superiority over milk. The state socked them with a $20,000 fine for restitution to residents who had bought the product and for costs of the investigation.

The Food and Drug Administration also went after Meadow Fresh for its "exaggerated claims that they were nutritionally equal or superior to milk, contained no cholesterol and were suitable as substitutes for cow's milk and mother's milk."[4] The FDA sometimes gets it right.*

The American Academy of Pediatrics has stated that coconut oil imitation milks should not be the major caloric source for infants and young children.**

As you might expect, the dairy industry has come out strong against imitation milks, pointing out the nutritional inferiority of the imitations. If I had to choose between the dairy industry's heated and homogenized milk and a vegetable oil—GRAS chemical combination, I would take the inferior milk. Don't get me wrong, I'm not taking the side of the National Dairy Association. We're talking about the lesser of evils.***

Robert E. Rich, Sr., the developer of the phony "cream" they inevitably serve you in America's fast food eateries, hopes that, "Someday you may have to go to the zoo to see a cow." Do you suppose Rich is biased? Did you ever read the label on one of those cute little "cream" cups? The main ingredients are sugar and coconut oil. The rest is sodium caseinate mono and diglycerides' di-

---

* Even a broken clock is right twice a day.
** These same pediatricians prescribe infant formulas with a coconut oil base. I guess they don't read labels. See Chapter IX.
*** I say pox on both their houses.

Nutrient Analysis of Meadow Fresh Imitation Milk Compared to Various Real Milks
(Per 8 Ounce Serving, Regular Dilution/Strength)

Nutrients	Claim (1) Meadow Fresh	(2) Analysis Of Meadow Fresh Plain Flavor	(2) Analysis Of Meadow Fresh Chocolate Flavor	(3) Whole Milk (3.3% Fat)	(3) 2% Milk (2% Fat)	(3) 2% Milk With Non-Fat Milk Solids Added (2% Fat)	(3) Human Milk	(3) Instantized Non-Fat Dry Milk
Calories	93	153	153	150	121	125	171	82
Carbohydrate (gm)	13	20.4	25.8	11.4	11.7	12.2	17.0	11.9
Protein (gm)	3.2	5.7	2.0	8.0	8.1	8.5	2.5	8.0
Fat (gm)	3	5	5	8	5	5	10.8	.16
Vitamin A (IU)	1000	895	605	307	500	500	593	539
*Calcium (mg)	150	132	63	291	297	313	79	280e

Riboflavin (mg)	.42	.26	.12	.40	.40	.42	.09	.39
Iron (mg)	N/A	.36	1.4	.12	.12	.12	.07	.07
Vitamin D (IU)	100	N/A	N/A	100	100	100	N/A	N/A
Thiamin (mg)	.09	N/A	N/A	.09	.10	.10	.03	.09

*Brog claims 200 in his "Defense of Meadow Farms."

Information From:

(1) Meadow Fresh product information sheet.

(2) State of Utah; Department of Agriculture; June 1, 1981.

(3) *Composition of Foods*: "Dairy and Egg Products; Raw, Processed, Prepared," Agriculture Handbook 8-1; USDA: Agriculture Research Service; #'s 01-077; 01-079; 01-080; 01-107. November 1976.

potassium phosphate, chemical flavors and chemical colors. That's the list of ingredients on Coffee-Mate from the Carnation Company, the home of contented cows.

Oski, in his anti-milk book[5] says, "In the not too distant future, milk may be so transformed that you won't be able to recognize it." (1977) He was certainly right on target with that prediction.

These powdered milk substitutes and even regular powdered milk cause an increase in cavities. They are deficient in the essential amino acid, lysine. A Penn State University research group fed lysine-deficient milk to laboratory rats. Rat teeth are quite similar to humans in their physiological and biochemical makeup. They developed rampant cavities.[6]

There's another phony milk you should know about. It's called UHT milk. The dairy industry is producing this one in an attempt to regain business lost to filled milk vegetable products and other junk beverages.

UHT stands for ultra high temperature. What it means is that milk has been heated to such a high temperature that it is sterilized, just like surgical instruments. It can be shipped in unrefrigerated trucks—a tremendous savings to the dairymen. It will sit on a shelf, unrefrigerated, for months without spoiling. The reason it won't spoil is because no self-respecting bug will eat it. Bugs are smart. They like fresh food with nutrient value, not steamcleaned pseudo food.

"Steam cleaning" is not just a figure of speech. That's exactly what they do. The method is described in Dairy Record, which is the national news magazine of the dairy industry, "Direct steam ...is added directly into the product, or... the product is added to the steam." They blast the milk at a temperature of 300°F! No wonder it will keep without refrigeration. Plaster of Paris will keep the same way.*

---

*It's probably about as good for you.

But the consumer is being oversold on the keeping qualities of this stuff. Once the package is opened, it will eventually spoil. It won't turn into safe, sour milk. But, like pasteurized milk, it will become rancid. Prediction: A false sense of security, caused by over-selling of UHT's keeping properties will lead to outbreaks of food poisoning.

The dairy industry has now refined its counterattack against the imitation milk invasion. You fight fire with fire, so why not junk milk against junk imitation of milk?

Their new junk food product called Sip-Ups can sit on the shelf for months without refrigeration just like the imitation powdered milks. It is composed of the new UHT, superheated milk which is low-fat (See Chapter III about low-fat milk). It contains various imitation flavors such as vanillin and, of course, lots of sugar.

The adverse effect on your health caused by even moderately heating milk was known over fifty years ago. In 1930 a fascinating article was published by the First International Congress of Microbiology meeting in Paris.[7] Dr. Paul Kouchakoff of the Institute of Clinical Chemistry, Lausanne, Switzerland, reported on the way the blood reacts to foods. Each food has a critical temperature above which the blood will react in a protective way by increasing the number of white blood cells. They are soldiers coming to defend against a lethal foreign invader.

Dr. Kouchakoff determined that the critical temperature above which milk becomes recognized by the white cells of the blood as an enemy of the body is 191°F. *UHT milk is heated to 300°F.*

They also add "vitamin" D3. Vitamin D isn't really a vitamin but a steroid hormone like cortisone. D3, used in Sip-Ups, has been proven to be an "angio-toxic risk factor."[8] That means, in plain language, that "vitamin" D can mess up your arteries and cause arteriosclerosis, which leads to high blood pressure, heart attacks, strokes and kidney failure.*

---

* The scientific name for D3 is cholecalciferol. You wouldn't want to feed it to a guest unless you owed him a lot of money.

Can you guess what the main thrust of the advertising for this sugar-coated, angiotoxic risk factor is? Better nutrition for your kids!

What can you do? Avoid these man-made products. Educate your children about the importance of eating fresh food, as uncooked as possible, and set an example for them. You can make a good start by feeding your family raw certified milk. If it's illegal in your state, do something about it.

REFERENCES

1. Food Processing, October, 1981.

2. Crest Foods Technical Bulletin #300.

3. Case #3 AN-81-5589.

4. FDA Talk Paper, Feb. 2, 1982.

5. Don 't Drink Your Milk, Oski & Bell, 1977.

6. Los Angeles Times, April 16, 1976.

7. Lee Foundation for Nutritional Research, Milwaukee, Wisconsin, 53201, Reprint #101.

8. American Journal Clin. Nut. 32: January, 1979, pp.58.

Chapter IX

UDDER PERFECTION

"It's a bit late in the day to introduce the idea now, but almost any mammal's milk would be easier to modify than cow's milk. Pig's milk is actually nearest to human milk. Camel milk and mare's milk have a better balance for humans. Sheep's milk is okay and so is goat's milk. Reindeer milk would be a bit fat, dog's milk a bit thin. Now, otter's milk could be just right. Perhaps we should look into it." ...(M. Bateman, 1975)

After delivery, the first milk of the human mother is called colostrum. It has a peculiar lemon yellow appearance. It is very high in antibodies so as to provide the newborn baby protection against infection. After the first few weeks, the milk turns to a more characteristic color for human milk, which is a bluish, thin liquid. This is often alarming to the mother expecting it to look like cow's milk.

The colostrum is extremely high in antibodies, especially IGA and lactoferrin, the primary function of which is to protect the baby from infection. It is *the* milk and *the only* milk that is perfect for the newborn baby.

The actual secretion of milk from the breast does not usually start until the baby starts sucking on the breast. A remarkable hormonal system begins to work. With the sucking of the breast there is stimulation of the anterior pituitary gland in the brain which excretes the hormone prolactin, and the prolactin in turn stimulates the breast to produce milk. The importance of this hormone is illustrated by the fact that women with diseases of the pituitary gland may be unable to produce milk because of the undersecretion of prolactin.[1]

A newborn baby has a very strong sucking reflex which should be taken advantage of by putting the baby on the breast immediately after birth. During assisted delivery, if the obstetrician's finger accidentally enters the baby's mouth, the baby will immediately start sucking on the finger.

Unfortunately, in hospital deliveries, the custom has been immediately to separate the mother from the baby, so the strong initial sucking reflex is not utilized to help the mother bring on her milk. This early sucking after delivery and before removal of the placenta has profound hormonal effects and should by all means be taken advantage of. Placental separation is facilitated by prolactin secretion. Prolactin is a built-in birth control system, for as long as the baby is sucking at the breast, prolactin is produced and the mother will not become pregnant.* It also helps water conservation and has a tranquilizing effect on the mother.

Another hormone, oxytocin, is important in the actual secretion of the milk. Without proper oxytocin production from the posterior pituitary gland, there is an inability of the milk to be "let down." Essentially, the milk will become unavailable.

Emotional factors in breast feeding are extremely important, and it is well known that a mother's milk can completely dry up if the mother becomes upset. The release of epinephrine causes a constriction of blood vessels around the breast which keeps circulating oxytocin from reaching the target organ. Conversely, from a positive point of view, a woman's milk will often flow if the mother sees her baby or even hears it cry. Even the thought of nursing can cause the "letting down" of milk. Modern medicine tends to interfere with all the natural processes necessary for the complicated hormonal interaction leading to the letting down of milk and the actual secretion of milk. The Western practice of giving comple-

---

*This doesn't *always* work, so don't say I didn't warn you.

mentary bottle feedings is only to be deplored as it decreases the child's appetite which leads to a diminished sucking reflex. A diminished sucking reflex causes a diminution in the prolactin secretion causing less production of milk, which may lead the mother to think she is inadequate. This in turn leads to anxiety, which leads to depression of oxytocin. The feeding of bottle milk between breast feeding may confuse the baby, as the sucking mechanism is entirely different between breast and artificial bottle feeding.

The baby should be immediately put on the breast following delivery, intermittent bottle feeding should be discouraged, and mother and baby should be kept together at all times to encourage feeding on demand. This will lead to a healthy baby, a quick recovery by the mother, and little need for the pediatrician.

The baby formula companies and the National Dairy Association have discouraged breast feeding through subtle advertising and clever propaganda. The National Dairy Association's animal pictures for children are a good example of anti-breast propaganda. Entitled "We All Like Milk," it is a set of twelve color prints of animals. It is indeed attractive and appealing to children. But study of these photographs reveals some rather interesting points.

First, it should be noted that animals do indeed like mother's milk, but in only one of the twelve photographs is there actually a scene of a baby nursing the mother. Some of the pictures show adult animals without any baby in the picture at all. The implication is that these adult animals drink milk, which of course, they do not. After all, the title of this children's picture series is "We All Like Milk," meaning the animals pictured.

Out of the twelve photos, the only one showing a baby actually nursing at the mother's breast is a picture of a very drab and filthy Polish ox, an essentially extinct animal. This leaves the impression that breast feeding also is extinct, and only a crummy animal like the Polish oxen would ever entertain such a yucky habit. The only reference to milk in the information provided on the back of the picture is the question, "What is the baby doing?" The answer is, by implication: He's engaging in an obscene, dirty, extinct habit practiced only by filthy animals. You think I'm a little paranoid? Send two bucks to the National Dairy Association, Chicago, Illinois 60606, and ask for a copy of "We All Like Milk." Decide for yourself.

Babies At The Breast
(From the Spiney Anteater to the Blue Whale)

The way the good Lord (or the Big E—evolution, if you are so inclined) has designed the feeding and care of the newborn in the mammalian world is truly fascinating and almost endless in variety.

The kangaroo illustrates one of the most amazing examples of the way nature provides for the young. The tiny (bean-sized), blind baby kangaroo, called a joey, is born while still a small fetus. This occurs at about four weeks gestation at which time the tiny little fetus actually migrates up the mother's abdominal wall to her pouch where it becomes firmly attached to one of the nipples in the pouch. It is then termed a "mammary-fetus." This is truly one of nature's most amazing feats of gestation and nourishing. The fixation of the joey to the teat is so firm as to be almost inseparable. There is a ridge in the hard palate of the joey and an indentation on the tongue which facilitates the taking of the teat into the mouth and fusing it directly into the little embryo's throat which makes a true umbilical cord-like continuity of feeding and attachment which is as secure as a true umbilical cord. The milk of the kangaroo mother, incidentally, is quite pink in color, contains no lactose, and is very high in protein.

The growth of the little embryo is phenomenally fast, as he grows from a weight of fifty milligrams when entering into the pouch to fifty grams in fifty days.

This is not the end of the remarkable story of the kangaroo nursing phenomenon. In addition to the neonatal joey at the nipple just described, the preceding offspring, known as a "young at foot," spends most of his time out of the mother's pouch hopping around the neighborhood. However, if he becomes alarmed, he can return temporarily to the pouch and suckle from a different nipple than a joey, *obtaining milk of an entirely different concentration appropriate for his particular age of development!* The next fertilized egg is not passed down and out the exterior of the kangaroo mother as long as the joey is attached to her teat. The egg simply remains dormant until the joey comes loose from her teat, at which time the next ovum will begin to develop.

Mammals are different in that they are the only animals in which the post-embryonic young is solely dependent on food supplied by the mother's body. The German word for mammal is very apt, saugetier, which means sucking animal. The word "mammal" comes from the Latin meaning breast.

In all but the higher animals this nursing process is purely instinctive. But with man and chimpanzees it has to be at least partly learned. Gunther reported that two chimpanzees born in a zoo to a non-wild mother were reported to have died of starvation from a failure of the mother to nurse. A non-wild female gorilla in a California game reserve was successfully assisted in nursing by the use of films showing mothers nursing their young during her pregnancy; she nursed very successfully. Higher forms of mammalian animals have learned a definite group behaviour which protects the female during her pregnancy, during her labor, and during the nursing period. Elephants, dolphins, and baboons all have group behaviour which illustrates this.

Predators, animals who usually do not have to worry about being eaten by other animals, have young who are relatively immature and require rather long nursing. Species with well-hidden nests or burrows, such as rabbits and mice, also have a very long period of dependency of the babies on the mother for nursing.

Animals which are preyed upon, and so need to be able to run almost immediately after birth, have very short gestation periods and are born nearly mature. Dolphins, whales, seals, deer, etc., are born almost mature and either suckle standing on their feet, or in the case of dolphins and whales, while swimming with their mother. Man is unique among the mammals in that he has a very long gestation period, has a very immature newborn incapable of doing anything for himself, and has a long period of breast feeding. The newborn human is one of the few mammals not able to even reach the breast without help from the mother. In most species the babies themselves instinctively find the breast with the mother simply lying in a passive role. As pointed out by Gunther, a little piglet at birth, apparently compelled by smell, scrambles around over its mother's legs until it reaches an unseen nipple entirely without the help of the mother.

In general, the protein content of the milk varies with the rate of growth of the particular offspring. This is known as Bunge's Law. As an example, the horse, with two percent protein in the milk, takes sixty days to double the birth weight. The rabbit, with twelve percent protein in the milk, doubles the birth weight in only six days. In other words, the growth rate is directly proportional to the amount of protein in the breast milk. The protein concentration is also related to the frequency with which the mother feeds her offspring. Human breast milk, for instance, has one of the lowest protein concentrations of all mammals, and feeding is fairly frequent. By contrast, the protein milk of the rabbit is so high that she feeds her offspring only once in a twenty-four hour period. The mouse, with a very low solute milk, in contrast, spends about eighty percent of its time feeding its young.

There is a great variability in the fat concentration of milk. Those animals requiring a lot of protection from extreme cold have a very high concentration of fat, whereas those who do not require this have a very low concentration of fat. For example, elephant milk contains only twenty percent fat, while the milk of the blue whale is fifty percent fat. Its newborn, which is twenty feet in length, lives in the cold water of the Arctic Sea and requires a great deal of protection from the cold temperatures. Those animals feeding on a high-fat milk grow at a prodigious rate. The whale pup increases his weight from forty to four hundred pounds in the first month of life!

The milk of one mammal is often entirely unfit for the young of another species. Some nutritionists feel very strongly about this in relation to cow's milk and human babies. Certainly, as we will see later in this chapter, cow's milk is a poor substitute for human breast milk.

Some examples of this incompatibility of various mammalian milks will illustrate the need for giving serious attention to those nutritionists who consider cow's milk incompatible with human infant digestion. The walrus, for example, produces a milk which contains very little lactose, and cow's milk, which is four percent lactose, causes severe diarrhea in the newborn walrus. Because of this, if the baby walrus is reared in captivity without mother's milk, he is fed a formula of blended raw fish and whipping cream. Baby kangaroos brought up on cow's milk develop cataracts. They lack the enzyme to metabolize lactose.

The spiney anteater is another example of the wondrous ways that nature provides for feeding the young. The mother anteater lays one single egg which is lodged in a deep depression in the mother's abdominal wall similar to a kangaroo pouch, except much smaller. The skin of the mother closes completely over the egg. The tiny young, about one inch long, hatches from this egg and remains in this little pouch in which there are two teats from which to feed. There the baby spiney anteater stays until it becomes too spiney for comfort.

The baby duck-billed platypus, which is an egg-laying mammal, comes into the world facing a seemingly impossible task. The newborn have to lick milk droplets from special hairs on the mother's belly. The New Guinea spiney anteater also has a precarious nursing system. Mother's milk simply pools in a crease in her belly and it's every anteater baby for himself. If the milk is spilled, then they do without.*

The blue whale calf would appear to have a problem in that he cannot stay underwater very long. He has to suck under water to get his nourishment. This predicament has been solved by a system in which a very highly concentrated milk (50% fat), which is basically cream, is pumped very rapidly into the baby which can then surface for air.

The Hokkaido monkey of northern Japan has an interesting breast feeding pattern as reported in Jelliffee's excellent book on human breast milk. Jelliffee is, in turn, reporting from Helsing (1976). Monkeys are born in the spring and are suckled at the breast until autumn. At that time the mother leaves the young to fend for themselves, eating wild berries and other edible material they can find near their nest. The mother goes out and eats voraciously to prepare her physiological winter store of food. When winter comes, and the heavy snow covers the ground, consequently making it very difficult for the young to find food, the infants go back to the breast and feed again until spring. Although the mother has not lactated for a number of months in this unusual situation, lactation starts again, and the monkeys are breast-fed until spring approaches.

Human milk is extremely complex and biologically different from any other milk. The milk of the goat, buffalo, reindeer, yak, camel, and even the horse have been used for feeding human children. But cow's milk is by far most common around the world, being used as the pro-

---

* The baby numbat doesn't have it easy either, but you probably don't care about the numbat.

tein base in most infant formulas. There are marked differences between the milk of the human and the milk of the cow, especially in the protein and fat content.

Human milk will vary according to the age of the infant and can even vary at different times of the day, and at different seasons of the year as the human breast will adjust to the baby's needs. So it will always be impossible to construct a milk formula from cows (or any other animal) that can equal a mother's milk. A fixed concentration of the various ingredients in a formula is not the physiological way, as a baby's needs are constantly changing. The human breast is smart enough to figure out what changes are needed. Man is not.

The Remarkable "White Blood" of Mother's Early Milk

The human newborn has been called by scientists an "exterogestate foetus," (a foetus outside the womb) because the baby is born just as helpless as he was in the mother. Even baby puppies have the ability to root around and find the mother's nipple, but the human baby must be placed on it. The human breast serves as an umbilical cord for the newborn, still foetus-like, baby so that the mother can continue to provide *life forces** essential to survival in a world loaded with menacing bacterial, viral, and fungal enemies. Her milk is an almost perfect shield against these predators.

In many ways the mother's early milk, called colostrum, acts as an antibiotic and is remarkably similar to blood in its content. In the *Koran* breast milk is referred to as "white blood." Murrilo and Goldman demonstrated in 1970 that human milk is indeed a very live fluid with very active enzymes, hormones, and cells just as in regular blood.

Mother's milk, because of its composition of enzymes, various blood cells, and antibodies, practically

---

*Not available in junk milk.

guarantees the infant against serious infection early in life, even in a poor environment where disease is rampant. The "bifidus factor" in human milk, for instance, facilitates the growth in the intestine of lactobacillus bifidus which has a protective effect on the young intestine. It stops the growth of undesirable organisms, such as E. coli, which can be fatal.

The intestinal bacterial population in babies fed on breast milk is very different from that of babies fed on cow's milk. The breast-fed baby's intestine is colonized mainly with the harmless lactobacillus bifidus, mentioned above, whereas the bottle-fed baby's intestine is populated primarily by gram negative bacteria which can cause serious illness. The following chart (Gotheforb) illustrates this critical difference.

Type of Bacteria	Breast-fed Infants	Bottle-fed Infants
Lactobacillus Bifidus	Dominant	Present in small numbers
Enterococci (A disease-causing organism)	Present in small numbers	Present in large numbers
E. Coli (A dangerous organism)	Usually present in small numbers	Constantly present in varying numbers, often dominant
Gram Negative Anaerobes (very dangerous organisms)	Mostly absent	Constantly present, sometimes in large numbers

You get the idea of how utterly ridiculous it is for the chemist to attempt to duplicate mother's milk with cow milk when you consider the incredible complexity of mother's milk, which includes not only the factors thus

far mentioned, but an amazing array of immunoglobulins, lysozyme bifidus factor, and nutrient carrier
proteins such as lactoferrin, and others, which literally
starve out enemy bacteria in the baby's intestinal tract.
The initial colostrum of milk shoots a large bolus of immunoglobulin into the baby to give it super protection
from infection. After a few days, as the needs become
less, the concentration of immunoglobulin falls off. The
immunoglobulin, IGA, absolutely essential for the baby
to resist disease, is present in only small amounts in cow
milk and is non-existent in "formula." The IGA in human
milk is one-hundred times more concentrated than in
cow's milk. The breast is actually a factory for this and
other important protective immunoglobulins.

The bifidus factor, first identified by Gyorgy, is extremely important. It facilitates the growth of the lactobacillus bifidus which checks the growth of undesirable
and dangerous organisms. Mother's milk contains forty
times as much of this important factor as cow milk.

An important enzyme, lysozyme, is a powerful antibiotic. Mother's milk has a lysozyme concentration approximately five thousand times greater than cow's milk.
Some cultures, instinctively aware of the antibiotic effect
of milk, have used it for such things as eye infections by
using the mother's milk as eye drops.*

The mother's milk produces interferon, which protects the baby against herpes virus, an antistaphlococcus
factor which protects the baby from the dreaded staph infection, anticholera factor, and also antibodies against ty-
phus. "Formula" contains none of these.

Another remarkable protective mechanism of the
human breast is the diathelic phenomenon. The diathelic
mechanism is a wonder of nature. The breast is stimulated by bacteria introduced at the teat by the baby. The
bacteria travel up the teat into the breast tissue, causing
an immediate reaction with the formation of antibodies,

---

*It works.

which can then be found back in the mother's milk within eight hours. If the mother is healthy, this is a practically fool-proof system of protection for the baby.

Klaus has stated it well, "The mother does not serve merely as a passive transmitter of immunity. Instead, the mammary gland is able to react to the microbes brought to it by the infant and respond with a fast production of specific antibody... The mammary gland is an exocrine reticuloendothelial gland which is 'lend leased' functionally to the infant at a time when his own reticuloendothelial system is inadequate."

The blood-like cellular composition of breast milk, mentioned above, is in itself another remarkable army designed to protect the newborn baby. The primary cell seen in the human milk is the macrophage. It dashes around squirting lysozyme at dangerous bacteria found in the intestine. It fires lactoferrin at the enemy, destroying yeast and other dangerous organisms by literally giving them an iron deficiency, rendering them impotent. These large cells, the macrophages, move around freely. As well as firing their special chemicals at unwanted organisms, they can also eat them. Another cell found in the blood and also found in the breast is called the lymphocyte. They produce inteferons and immunoglobulins to aid in the war against infection.*

A host of diseases attack the newborn bottle-fed baby which affect the breast-fed baby little or none at all. Among these are epidemic infectious diarrhea of the newborn, acute necrotizing enterocolitis, otitis media, septicemia, and others. *All of these diseases can be prevented, and usually cured, simply by the use of fresh, human breast milk.*

---

* Fantastic! How can the Mead Johnson Company, with their coconut oil formulas, compete with a system like that?

A typical example of the terrible havoc that can be unleashed in a person's life by improper feeding is the story of my patient, David Mishap (name fictitious—story real).

David was put on a formula immediately after an uneventful birth. He was sent home on this formula and in two weeks was back in the hospital because of severe incompatibility with the formula. David was placed in a room adjoining the pediatric intensive care unit. He thus was exposed to some lethal bacteria and ended up getting both streptococcus and staphlococcus infections. He was sent home with the infections unrecognized, and in a very short period of time the staph and strep infections had spread through the entire Mishap family.

This unlucky child experienced nothing but chronic illness during his entire childhood. He became a misfit in his class and eventually turned to drugs. David dropped out of high school. He has not been able to hold a job for any length of time. He is now twenty-one years old, is 5′ 8″ tall, and weighs one hundred-twenty pounds. All of his problems are attributable to a very sickly childhood, secondary to his chronic infections, starting at age one month, and from which he never completely recovered. He is a semi-invalid, unable to support himself, and disappointed in life in general. *All of this misery and expense probably could have been avoided if the child had been breast-fed from day one.*

There is a reason why breast-fed babies develop faster than bottle-fed ones. Dr. Michael Klagsbrun of Harvard has discovered a new growth factor in human colostrum.[2] None of the baby formulas contain this growth factor.*

In Russia, a mother is given a four-month maternity leave to establish a breast-feeding routine. When she returns to work, the baby receives care at a nursery where the mother works. Every three hours she may take a nursing break.**

---

* For the scientific reader: This factor is a mitogen that stimulates DNA synthesis.

** I hate communism, but by God they are right on this one.

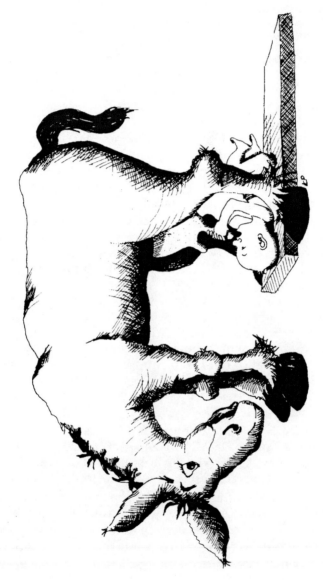

French Mothers, Using Donkeys, Used to do it This Way.

Producers of baby formula based on pasteurized cow's milk are fond of showing charts that would indicate that human milk and their "formula" are "more or less" the same. They list on their beautiful full-color brochures for mothers the comparative fat content. The fat content for human milk is 4.5 grams per 100 cc's, and for formula, SMA for instance, it is 3.6 grams per 100 cc's—not a great difference.

But, things are not always as they appear. Examination of the fat of the two milks shows them to be entirely different as to quality and kind. The levels of the essential polyunsaturated fatty acids are far greater in breast milk, especially linoleic acid which is seven to eight times greater. The fat used in commercial formula is coconut oil, a 95% saturated, indigestible fat suitable only for soap manufacture. The pasteurization process alters the fat further, making it even less digestible.

The vital chemical development of the brain is dependent on the proper concentrations of arachidonic and docadexaenoic fatty acids. These two important fatty acids are present in much lower concentrations in cow's milk formula. This may have tremendous import on the "brain pool" of our nation. We may, in fact, be draining our brain resources by dosing our babies with coconut oil[3].

A proper supply of cholesterol is extremely important for the infant. Cholesterol is necessary for the development of the enzyme systems of the body and is absolutely essential for proper development of the central nervous system. Human milk has a much higher cholesterol level than cow's milk. Most of the baby formulas are even lower in cholesterol because of their vegetable base.

Even baby formula, as bad as it is, may be safer than homogenized milk. Studies done in New Zealand revealed that babies raised on homogenized milk, compared to infant formula, were much more likely to become anemic due to blood in their stools. (Fifty-eight percent of the babies fed homogenized milk had blood in their stools.)

The homogenized milk babies also had a significantly higher blood cholesterol level. At the end of five
years these babies were tested again. They found that the
homogenized milk babies still had a higher cholesterol
level than the babies that were fed formula.

As we mentioned, babies need a high cholesterol intake
for proper brain development. But the cholesterol must be
in a natural state, as in mother's milk, so that it can be properly metabolized by the central nervous system. You want it
in the brain, not floating around in the blood.

Triglycerides are the main constituents of milk fat.
They have to be broken down in the presence of the enzyme lipase for digestion. Pasteurized cow's milk formula contains no lipase, whereas human milk is rich in
lipase. Consequently, human milk fat is very efficiently
digested, and formula is not.

The disease hypocalcemia of the newborn illustrates
the extreme importance of breast milk feedings. The palmitic acid of human milk is of a different chemical character from the palmitic acid of cow's milk. The
pasteurized cow's milk palmitic acid is precipitated by
calcium in the intestinal tract and is excreted as calcium
palmitate soap. This causes a loss of fat, and even more
important, a loss of calcium. A low calcium state and
hypocalcemia with convulsions may result.

It would appear, on analysis, that cow's milk is superior to human milk, as it contains three times as much
protein. The opposite is true, as the protein in cow's milk
is eighty-two percent casein. Casein causes a curd in the
stomach that is tough and rubbery as opposed to the soft
curd from human milk. Cow's milk, especially if pasteurized, is much less digestible in the delicate digestive system of the baby, and if overfeeding happens, an actual
milk blockage called lactobezoar can occur.[4]*

---

* A lactobezoar is like a baseball. You couldn't pass it and neither can
  your baby.

The differences between human milk and cow's milk formula go much deeper. Closer examination of the enzyme content of the two milks shows even more drastic differences of a highly technical nature. One of these differences illustrates the complexity of human milk and the futility of trying to duplicate it.

The milk enzyme lactoferrin causes a binding of iron in the baby's intestinal tract which makes this iron unavailable to harmful bacteria in the newborn baby's intestine. This in a sense starves the microorganisms, makes them "anemic," and therefore ineffective as far as causing gastrointestinal problems to the baby. But the infant formulas based on pasteurized cow's milk are usually "iron enriched" and contain no lactoferrin. The baby is in double jeopardy in that lactoferrin is not present, and iron is added to the milk which may enrich the unwanted bacteria. This may be a factor in so-called "milk intolerance" or "milk allergy."

On the question of vitamins, there is no doubt that human milk is a perfect vitamin combination for the baby, and no additional vitamins need be given. Pasteurized cow milk preparations may appear superficially to contain more or less the right amounts of the various vitamins. But investigation has shown some of them, Vitamin B12 for instance, to be present in a different form than in human milk and therefore not absorbable.

It would appear from the formula literature that breast milk and cow milk contain equal amounts of zinc, a very important nutrient to the young. But this also turns out to be more apparent than real, as the zinc from cow milk is not readily absorbed. Breast milk contains a zinc binding factor which favors proper absorption. There is a zinc deficiency disease known as acrodermatitis enteropathica. Acrodermatitis rarely occurs in the breast-fed infant.

Even the rate of breathing is different in babies fed on breast milk as compared to bottle feeding, and *this is true even if the breast milk itself is fed out of a bottle.* So the human teat also serves an important purpose.[5]

The message is clear: Breast is best. Mother's milk is more nutritious, anti-infective, contraceptive, and vastly more economical. The only milk that a young baby should receive is that which has been run, unpasteurized, through the mother.

The Baby Formula Diseases

Cow's milk formula feeding has become the norm in all western countries. The majority of people, both medical and non-medical, seem to think there is little difference in the eventual outcome, whether the child is breast-fed or fed pasteurized cow milk formula. The possible long term effects of artificial feeding had not been properly investigated or brought into focus until Jelliffee & Jelliffee' brought all the research together in their book *Human Milk in the Modern World.*[6]

Many studies of Western society have shown there is a definite tendency toward obesity among bottle-fed babies. In one study in Laborador, Canada, for instance, seventy percent of children under one year of age were obese. In the poorer countries, formula is almost certain to be diluted to a minimal level of nourishment because of the cost, leading to semi-starvation. In the more affluent countries, the opposite happens wherein the mother will make the formula more concentrated, thinking she is giving her baby extra nourishment. This leads to caloric overdose and, because of the high concentration of the formula, often leads to thirst, which in turn leads to the baby demanding more formula, creating a vicious cycle leading to obesity. The healthy human breast, on the other hand, regulates the baby's need to an incredible degree.

Tracey and others have demonstrated that the obese, bottle-fed baby is more subject to illness than the breast-fed baby. Even after bottle feeding has stopped in early childhood, the child denied the breast is more subject to illness. Respiratory infections and skin diseases are far more common in these bottle-fed, obese children.

The problem of bottle-feeding obesity is extremely serious, as many studies have now shown that the malady will continue into adult life, leading to permanent obesity with all of its concurrent physical risks. Eid demonstrated that eighty percent of obese children are also obese in adult life. It is well known that obesity is one of our major health problems. It may well stem from cow's milk bottle feeding from birth.

Iron deficiency anemia is far less common in breast-fed babies. The iron content of breast milk, and cow's milk as well, is low. However, the iron needs of the bottle-fed infant are higher, probably due to intestinal micro hemorrhages, which can deplete the baby's iron stores. Iron supplementation is always needed in the bottle-fed baby whereas it is not needed in the breast-fed baby.

Cow's milk has a different electrolyte (minerals) and protein content than human milk, and babies fed on modified cow's milk formula are reported to have a rather high level of urea. Urea is a breakdown product of protein, and in abnormal concentrations can put a heavy load on the baby's immature kidneys. Although it has not been proven, this may be a factor in adult hypertension and kidney disease. The excess sodium can cause the same kidney problems and possible brain damage in addition.

Fatty acids and calcium from cow milk combine to form insoluable soaps, making the calcium unavailable for absorption. This is the major reason why the stools of breast-fed babies are entirely different in appearance and odor from those of bottle-fed babies. This condition can be so serious that convulsion and death occur because of low blood calcium level. These low calcium, high phosphate, bottle-fed babies with "neonatal hypocalcemia" can also die of heart failure. This deadly syndrome simply does not occur in breast-fed babies.

The premature baby is almost assured of bad health, at least during childhood, if fed cow's milk baby formula. The amino acids in cow's milk are entirely different from that of human milk and the premature infant simply cannot metabolize it properly. The important amino acid, cystine, is of very low concentration in cow's milk. It is absolutely essential for the survival and good health of premature babies. Premature babies do not have the enzyme cystothianase in their livers and consequently cannot change other amino acids to the essential cystine. Mature infants usually have this enzyme and can convert the amino acids in cow's milk to cystine. The long term effects of feeding these highly vulnerable premature children cow's milk formula is devastating and permanently damaging. Learning disabilities caused by neurological damage from the ingestion of the high concentration of unassimilatable amino acids can lead to lifelong intellectual crippling. Certainly our brain resources, our "intellectual pool," is the most valuable commodity of our nation, and it is entirely possible that we are having a "brain drain" from this undesirable approach to infant feeding. As Dr. Royal S. Copeland once said, "The measure of a civilization is the fate of its babies."

Dyslexia, learning disabilities, and all the array of central nervous system problems we see today in children may be related to the abandonment of the breast. Frances Broad did a study in New Zealand in 1971 on the devastating effect that bottle feeding has on speech and learning.[7] It should have shocked American pediatricians into a campaign against bottle feeding.* Broad hypothesized that factors influencing the development of the sucking response could possibly have an effect on improving the muscles required for speech, including the tongue. Her findings were of enormous importance to parents, teachers, pediatricians, and speech therapists.

---

*But who reads the New Zealand Medical Journal?

Eighty-six percent of breast-fed boys had clear speech by the age of six, whereas only *forty-eight percent* of bottle-fed boys had clear speech at six years of age.* Only seven weeks of breast feeding was necessary to avoid the speech handicap.

Broad's major findings:

1. There is a distinct relationship between breast feeding and clear speech in the male child.
2. Breast feeding is associated with improved tonal quality in both sexes, but with a more marked improvement in the case of the male child.
3. *Improved speech is associated with improved reading ability.***

The disease acrodermatitis enteropathica is a good example of how things are not always as they appear. W.S. Gilbert said in H.M.S. Pinafore:

"Things are seldom what they seem,
Skim milk masquerades as cream."

Promoters of cow milk formula are quick to point out the similarity between cow milk and human milk rather than the differences. The zinc level of cow's milk and human milk is virtually the same, three to five milligrams per 100 cc's. But the assimilation of the zinc is an entirely different matter. The disease acrodermatitis enteropathica, which is fatal if not treated, appears to be a zinc deficiency caused by the zinc in cow's milk simply not being assimilated into the baby's metabolism. It is treated by administering zinc supplements or by simply feeding the babies mother's milk. As the cow's milk formula manufacturers continue to change their mixtures in

---

* Girls are not as affected speech-wise by bottle feeding.
** Now do you think it's important to breast feed your baby? If he can't read, he can't learn.

an attempt to emulate mother's milk, they end up solving one problem and creating others. These attempts at "humanizing" cow's milk have led to Vitamin B6 deficiency, linoleic acid deficiency, and hemolytic anemia due to Vitamin E deficiency.*

The udder folly of trying to duplicate mother's milk with a cow milk formula is illustrated by the comment from the Department of Health and Social Security of the United Kingdom in 1974, "Only by demineralization and addition of electrolytes can a food based on cow's milk be prepared which has the sodium concentration near to that of breast milk. But during this demineralization process all minerals are removed including known elements *and perhaps others as yet unknown.* When elements are replaced in the form of soluble inorganic salts, *there is no certainty that they are then present in physiologically ideal form.*" (Emphasis added.) In less scientific language: The minerals go in one end and come out the other.

There are many factors which led investigators to suspect that diseases in adults may very well have their etiology in formula feeding in infancy. Autopsies have shown that arteriosclerosis does indeed appear in bottle-fed children. Breast-fed babies simply do not have this bad beginning. The etiology of coronary artery disease, accelerated by the use of junk foods, probably does start with junk milk in childhood.

Contrary to propaganda put out by the American Medical Association, the American Heart Association, and other misguided groups, a high-cholesterol diet is probably protective against hardening of the arteries rather than causative. Human milk has a much higher level of cholesterol than cow milk as well as other factors, including more utilizable zinc, which helps to protect the baby against hardening of the arteries. There are, no doubt, many other factors involved, such as the use of

---

* Vitamin E was formerly called "a vitamin looking for a disease"—it found it.

chlorinated water in childhood, but "formula" appears to be a definite factor in early atherosclerosis.

Allergy to cow milk is a commonly recognized problem which usually starts in babyhood with the institution of cow milk formula. Multiple sclerosis and ulcerative colitis have also been associated with the use of cow milk. There is some evidence that unprocessed, that is raw unhomogenized milk, is much less likely to cause these syndromes.

One of the great enigmas of modern medicine is the "sudden infant death syndrome." It has become a leading cause of death in babies between one month and one year old in the modern world. Paradoxically, this syndrome appears to be almost unknown in many primitive societies. A highly significant study done by Tonkin in New Zealand reveals that of eighty-six babies dying with SID, only three were breast-fed. It would be interesting to know if the sudden infant death syndrome is increasing in those areas of the world previously untouched by cow milk formula.

Although a study of the sudden infant death syndrome has not proven a true bacteremia, that is, infection of the blood, it is known that there is a marked "immunity gap" when the child is fed cow milk rather than human milk. The breast-fed baby has built-in immunity from the mother's milk, whereas the newborn fed on cow's milk only has temporary immunity brought in by the mother's blood at birth. At about the time this temporary immunity wears off at three months of age, the incidence of sudden death goes up. If these babies were breast fed, these deaths simply would not occur. The cause of the sudden infant death syndrome is unclear, but breast feeding will avoid most cases.*

In advanced societies there are significant differences in the incidence of illness between breast-fed and bottle-fed infants. It amounts to many millions of dollars

---

*We covered this in more detail in Chapter III.

of income and energy lost every year. A study done by Wako of Japan revealed a 31.4% respiratory illness rate in bottle-fed babies as compared to only 16% for breast-fed. Cunningham, in his study, found respiratory infections, otitis media, vomiting, and diarrhea to be three times as common in bottle-fed babies in New York.

Dr. Randolph Paine of the University of Iowa studied 106 babies, forty of whom were breast-fed and the remaining 66 bottle-fed. He compared the method of feeding with the number of visits due to illness to the doctor's office. The breast-fed infants had an average of 1.6 visits to the doctor. The bottle-fed infants averaged 2.8.

A study done in 1981 at Massachusetts General Hospital reported on the incidence of viral infection of newborn babies which, the author suggested, could be avoided by "later delivery." What the author was saying was that the incidence of this disease was more common in premature babies. The significant omission in this report was that no mention was made as to whether these babies were breast-fed or bottle-fed. Undoubtedly, the whole syndrome could be avoided if all babies were breast-fed. This article reflects the total lack of knowledge and interest in breast feeding and its curative properties by most modern-day physicians. In fact a study in California revealed that over half of the pediatricians and obstetricians surveyed had never seen a baby breast fed either in their childhood or during their medical training.[8] An editorial in the Lancet, a prestigious British medical journal, came down hard on the pediatricians, "...having in effect abdicated their responsibilities in this field (they) must accept responsibility for the present state of affairs."

The psychological factors in breast feeding as compared to bottle feeding are difficult to measure. Many investigators feel there is a connection between the decrease in the ability to maintain loyalties over a period of time and the progressive destructive behavior seen in modern society as breast feeding has declined and bottle feeding has increased. One cannot help but notice the obsession that Western men have with the appearance of women's breasts. Is this related to the decline in breast feeding in Western civilization?

Nizel of Tufts University reported that decayed teeth were four times more common in pasteurized milk-fed babies as opposed to breast-fed babies.*

It is obvious to even a casual observer that the brace business has become a major industry in this country in the past fifty years. No one seems to question why a large percentage of children need braces, whereas fifty years ago they did not. Some would respond that the technology simply was not there, but the facts would belie this conclusion. Adults now fifty years or more of age certainly do not appear to have more crooked teeth than younger people. They, in fact, seem to have less. This severe malarrangement of teeth, due to abnormal development of the mouth and nasopharyngeal cavity, is due to the change from breast feeding to bottle feeding. The mechanics of breast feeding as compared to bottle feeding are entirely different and this affects the development of the entire oropharynx. It is probable that ninety-eight percent of the orthodontists would be put out of business if there was a general return to breast feeding. Dr. Weston Price proved that processed food, such as pasteurized milk, causes poor development of the facial bones which leads to a mouth too small for all the teeth.

The economic losses from bottle feeding as opposed to breast feeding are truly staggering. Jelliffee & Jelliffee point out just one tiny aspect of this problem:

"...In the USA, a bottle-fed baby uses about one hundred fifty tins of ready-to-feed formula at six months. With an estimated 3,000,000 births per annum in the USA, this implies not only the loss of large quantities of milk, but at the same time, the use of 450,000,000 usually non-recyclable tins, or about 70,000 tons of tinplate each year."

---

*See also Steinman rat studies on page 41.

To this could be added the cost of tons of bottles, plastic or glass, nipples, sterilizing equipment, possibly increased crime, skyrocketing costs of orthodontics, and doctor and hospital bills amounting to billions of dollars.

One of the very slick promotion pieces from the National Dairy Council entitled *Calcium Throughout the Life Cycle* makes some interesting comments concerning calcium in cow's milk and calcium in breast milk. One gets the impression from this booklet that there is some question as to whether the baby gets enough calcium through the breast. But the Dairy Council goes on to assure the reader, "Since the smaller quantity of calcium in human milk is balanced by increased absorption, breast feeding fulfills calcium needs."

This "damnation through faint praise" is entirely misleading. What the article does not say is that the only cases of neonatal hypocalcemia, low calcium in the blood, are found in pasteurized, cow's milk-fed and formula-fed infants.

The brochure goes on to state, "Throughout adolescence and early adult life an adequate intake of calcium enriched foods such as milk and milk products is necessary for complete mineralization of the skeleton." This is an exaggeration of the importance of milk and milk products. One hundred grams of milk, for instance, only supplies ten percent of the recommended daily allowance of calcium for adults. Calcium is readily available in a diet consisting of fresh fruits and vegetables which are not overcooked. I do not mean to imply that milk and dairy products cannot or should not supply a portion of calcium needs. But the question still must be answered as to how much of the calcium in a pasteurized homogenized product is really available? Are we seeing a vast number of patients with osteoporosis (thinning bones) because these so-called high-calcium dairy products do not have a calcium that is assimilable? There are many areas of the world where milk and dairy products in general are not in great use, and yet these people have no more osteoporosis or other diseases of low calcium than we do. Many have less. The Dairy Council booklet states that the calcium phosphorus ratio of 1.2 to 1.0 in pasteurized cow's milk is conducive to skeletal growth and favors calcium absorption into the bone. This is untrue. The calcium phosphorus ratio in cow's milk is not conducive to absorption. The excess of phosphate in pasteurized cow's milk actually diminishes the serum calcium level. More importantly, the enzymes necessary for the proper absorption of calcium have been destroyed by the pasteurization process. The booklet states, "Milk or other dairy products become dietary essentials if the calcium needs of the various age groups are to be met." Actually, the calcium needs of the individual can be met without ever drinking milk or eating milk products. But if you want to be assured of getting adequate calcium in your diet, drink a pint of *raw* milk every day.

The Great American Allergy Problem

Jelliffee has pointed out that a fully bottle-fed baby of three months of age consumes his own body weight in pasteurized cow's milk every week. Six grams per kg of cow's milk that the baby drinks is equivalent to seven quarts of milk per day for an adult! If the baby is allergic to components of pasteurized cow's milk, he is obviously getting a huge dose of the allergic components on a daily basis.

The incidence of allergy among breast-feeding babies is practically zero. It should be pointed out that the bottle milk we are talking about is pasteurized milk and pasteurized milk formula. The incidence of allergy to cow milk is greatly reduced when the milk is unprocessed, that is, raw and unhomogenized. But, as we have pointed out many times, there is no substitute for mother's milk. An example of the importance of mother's milk in avoiding allergy are the statistics from Kampala,

Uganda. This very busy urban hospital with one hundred pediatric beds, reported absolutely no food allergy in the one year of the study. The babies are breast fed in Kampala.

As long ago as 1934, fifty years ago, it was known that the incidence of allergic disease was seven times as common in bottle-fed babies.[9] The array of diseases associated with pasteurized cow's milk is truly staggering: otitis media, bronchial pneumonia, failure to thrive, diarrhea, anemia, gastroenteropathy, vomiting, malabsorption syndrome, atopic dermatitis, rhinitis, colitis, colic, anaphylactic shock, sudden infant death syndrome, and intussusception (a telescoping of the bowel). Various difficulties of adulthood including multiple sclerosis, coronary artery disease (heart attack), and ulcerative colitis, have been associated with cow's milk allergy in early childhood.

Immunoglobulin A (IGA) is not present in the intestinal canal of the newborn for six weeks. The IGA is extremely important, in fact essential, for avoidance of allergy in babies. But the mother's breast milk contains adequate amounts of IGA to protect the baby. Cow's milk does not have the all-important IGA, so as stated unequivocally by Jelliffee, "Feeding is the single most important approach to prophylaxis of allergy in infancy." Jelliffee goes on to recommend that absolutely no other foods be given to the infant for the first six months of life, that is nothing but breast milk to avoid these allergic problems. Jelliffee's opinion is reinforced by the work of Mellon, who proved, by using breast feeding for allergic infants, that he could reduce the incidence of allergy from forty-one percent to a mere seven percent.

It is worth emphasizing again that all of these studies to which we have referred involve the use of pasteurized milk, not unprocessed raw milk. The advantage of raw milk as a substitute for breast milk, when necessary, is discussed in another chapter.

Cavity formation in young babies is directly related to the type of milk the baby has been fed. Babies who are breast fed have considerably fewer cavities than babies who are bottle fed. Even if the child is breast fed for only three months, a study by Tank & Storvick revealed that these children had fifty percent fewer cavities than children fed on cow's milk. I told you more about this in Chapter III.

Severe deficiencies often occur in undeveloped countries where pasteurized cow milk formula has been foisted on the ignorant public. Scurvy (Vitamin C deficiency) and Vitamin A deficiency are the two most common. The problem goes beyond the home in that the same ignorance extends to the hospitals, the doctors, and the nursing personnel. One study in a third-world country showed that *eighty-seven percent* of the children admitted to the hospital were malnourished. The problem worldwide is mind-boggling. Estimates are that there is a total of 98.4 million children between birth and four years of age suffering from some form of malnutrition. Much of this malnutrition would be avoided by expelling Nestle, Borden, SMA, and other formula manufacturers from the various countries involved.

A group called Infant Formula Action is organizing a boycott of Nestle products in developing countries, demanding that this company stop the free distribution of formula in hospitals and that clinics stop the use of "Mother Craft Nurses" who promote formula use.*

Little understood but of great importance in controlling world population is "lactation amenorrhea." The secretion of prolactin hormone acts as a natural contraceptive, important in spacing children in poor countries. This natural spacing puts the children from one and one-half to two years apart. This contraceptive effect of breast feeding has been common knowledge in primitive tribes for hundreds and perhaps thousands of years, but it has not been accepted in modern society until very recently.

---

*Nestle agreed in 1984 to stop these practices.

The Eskimo women of twenty-five years ago breast fed their babies for as long as three years and conception only occurred two to four months after the cessation of breast feeding. The increase in birth rate in the Eskimo can be correlated with the proximity of their living quarters to the nearest trading center selling tinned milk. It is probably no exaggeration to say that a great deal of the world's present population problems can be laid on the shoulders of the commercial infant formula companies.

The incredible impact on the economy of a poor nation caused by the abandonment of breast feeding is seldom realized. Byrd pointed out that in Kenya there was an approximate eleven and one-half million dollar annual loss in breast milk *which is two-thirds of the National Health budget or one-fifth of the annual economic aid given to that country!** Multiply this by all of the disadvantaged countries of the world, and the cost is truly staggering. These cost figures do not even take into consideration the tremendous lack of brain development, chronic illness and associated medical costs, giving these nations a burden from which they can probably never recover. Or, at least, not until they recognize that commercial formula companies are one of their greatest enemies and not the great benefactors they pretend to be in their advertising.

It should be pointed out that these health problems of children and the birth rate situation also apply to the disadvantaged people in the more advanced countries. Although to a lesser degree, protein malnutrition and chronic disease caused by formula can be found in Harlem and Birmingham just as it can in Ghana and Bangledesh.

Baby Formula—Junk Food

The search for the perfect artificial mother's milk goes on, and, of course, it will never be found. The con-

---

* The loss is computed by determining how much formula had to be bought to replace breast milk not utilized for infant feeding.

fusing array of various "milks" available, each claiming to be superior, is truly remarkable. In 1974, a study by Ford of the thirty-two formula preparations in Europe showed that the difference in composition of these various milks was vast. Many of them were a dangerous mixture of animal and vegetable fats, including coconut oil. In the United States this trend toward polyunsaturated fats is perhaps even more extreme. Coconut oil is commonly used. I can assure you that the human breast does not contain any coconut oil, and, although good for making soap, it certainly is not designed for the delicate intestines of the newborn child. In restrained understatement Jelliffee says, "The nutritional effect of these changes are quite uncertain." What do the following have in common: Similac baby formula, Dove soap, Enfamil baby formula, Lifebuoy soap, and Meadow Fresh imitation milk?*

Recent investigations in Sweden have shown that the protein content of human milk is lower than we once thought. Which means, in all probability, that we have been overloading babies with excess protein in formula which contributes to kidney disease, allergies, high blood pressure, and a host of other diseases.

It is characteristic of man that he periodically has to rediscover the wheel. There is today, in industrialized countries, a quiet revolution going on as people go to natural methods in medicine and rediscover the breast. Unfortunately, the third-world countries are now facing the same onslaught by commercial baby formula people that the Western world faced fifty years ago. The formula companies are looking for new markets as they face a shrinking market in a more sophisticated Western world. This tragic exploitation of these ignorant people and the consequent abandonment of a great national resource, human milk, must be stopped.

Estrada, commenting in an editorial in the journal of the Philippine Medical Association, said, "Advertise-

---

*You guessed it. Coconut oil.

ments of cow's milk preparations bombard the population, especially the nursing mothers, from all quarters;
billboards, pictures, magazines, radio, and television, all
show in glowing color the sturdiness and attractiveness
of babies (and their mothers) if they use this or that product. This is such that it had been found, particularly in
developing countries, that artificial feeding becomes a
manifestation of status, used by those who belong to a
higher social level, and breast feeding is only for... the
lower strata of the population. "

The first experiment in medical manslaughter with
artificial milk as the weapon was probably the one in 1 g
12 when the Germans introduced bottle feeding to the
people of East Africa. The results were of course disastrous with a drastic increase in "intestinal catarrh" and infant death.

In Costa Rica over forty percent of infants are
weaned from the breast by age of four months. This is in
a country with extremely limited means of obtaining
wealth with no petroleum and an economy that is pretty
much at the mercy of world prices for agricultural products. In a small village in Mexico as high as ninety percent of babies were breast-fed until three months of age,
but in 1971 breast feeding had plummeted to about five
percent. Taken to the extreme, at the University of Western Nigeria at Ibadan, the babies are one hundred percent bottle-fed from birth.

The revolt against artificial feeding is due to a general reaction against modern technology and to an aware-
ness that anti-allergic, emotional and other factors are
very much involve d in breast feeding. There is a realization that doctors and other health professionals really
don't know what they are talking about when it comes to
infant feeding.

The promotion of junk milk formulas throughout the
world is done with tremendous advertising budgets. The
advertising promotion campaigns are pervasive, insidi-

ously anti-breast milk, extremely effective—and devastating to the health of the population of the poor countries. The food companies, mostly American, hand out many free samples, weight charts, and measuring tapes, calendars, and other paraphernalia with the company name usually on it. Company "milk nurses" or "mother craft nurses" have been utilized to promote formula. They work as trained nurses and do nursing assignments, but they are also the active sales representatives and promoters for the company by which they are employed.

In the poorer countries, these campaigns cause a drastic dislocation of the economy in that the natives, perceiving this as the epitome of modern life, abandon breast feeding to purchase the vastly inferior baby formula. This takes a large percentage of their monthly income, not to mention the tremendous increase in diseases of the children who become a burden on the already impoverished government. These campaigns are very similar to the ones used by the junk food industry to promote soda pop around the world and in the long run will probably be even more medically and economically disastrous.

This type of promotion, of course, goes on in our own country to even a greater extent, and these junk formulas are promoted among the medical profession incessantly. The companies take advantage of the fact that most doctors and nurses are largely ignorant on nutrition, so in a sense, the formula companies are playing on ignorance just as they do in developing countries. The American Medical Association and its journals, such as the pediatric journals, are almost entirely supported from funds contributed by the drug industry and the food industry. Without the advertising from the drug industry and the food industry, the American Medical Association and all its journals would simply collapse. Even if the doctors and nurses were more sophisticated on nutrition, how can they bite the hand that feeds them?

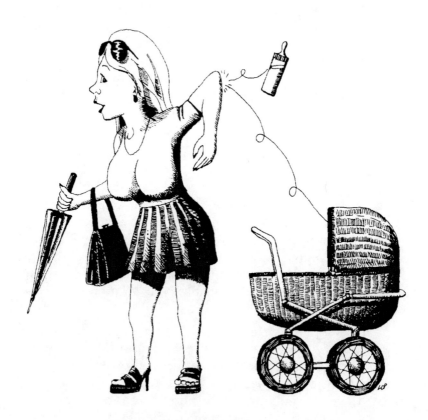

*The Babies of the World are Revolting Against
Artificial Feeding*

Economic Rape by Bottle Feeding

It is truly amazing that most of the world has turned away from breast milk in the face of actual starvation to take to nutritionally inferior bottle feeding. Jelliffee points out that perhaps we should not be really surprised that human milk has not been considered as a national resource in food by the bureaucratic planners, as it is not grown agriculturally or purchased in a can. In 1968 a United Nations Publication entitled *International Action to Avert the Impending Protein Crisis* made no mention whatsoever of human milk. Yet to supply cow's milk formula for all women with babies in India, for instance, would require the development of an additional herd of fourteen million milk-producing cows. This is clearly impossible and unnecessary when mother's milk is readily available even in malnourished women.

The cost of abandoning breast milk feeding, especially in underdeveloped countries, has been truly staggering. Not only do all the tons of breast milk have to be replaced with inferior cow's milk formula at great cost, but the incredible amount of disease to infants has to be treated with expensive medications, hospital facilities, doctors, nurses, and other personnel. Also the problem of birth control in these countries is made even worse by the simple fact that the loss of lactation means the loss of the natural contraceptive hormone which prevents pregnancy during active lactation. In one California city, it cost approximately three times as much to feed a baby ready-to-feed formula rather than spend the money for food for the mother which is converted to breast milk.[10] This difference in cost would be extremely important to families at the poverty level.

As an aside, it should be mentioned that along with the bad attitude toward breast feeding in the United States, can be added that doctors for years have given prospective mothers very bad advice concerning weight gain. Doctors have insisted for years that women carefully restrict their weight during pregnancy under the misconception that this would prevent hypertension and eclampsia (convulsions). Whichelow in 1975 showed that women who drastically reduced their calorie intake had immediate reduction in milk supply. Failure of lactation may be due, in part, to this bad medical advice.

The price of dried skim milk, the basic ingredient of most baby formulas, has quadrupled in the last few years. Although the price of food to the mother has of course risen, there has been no rise in cost of labor, packaging, or delivery in the maternal "milk factory." So the cost of breast feeding still remains about one-third the cost of formula.

One of the great scandals in international business today is the incredible "rip-off" of poor people around the world buying baby formula. The cost per day at six months of age for feeding a baby an adequate amount of baby formula would require sixty-three percent of the average Egyptian's wage. A ministry clerk in Malawi spends eighty percent of his salary to buy enough formula to feed his baby, whereas it is available for practically nothing right at the mother's breast. This is a truly pathetic swindle of innocent people.

The evidence from sound research indicating the superiority of breast milk over prepared cow milk formula is undisputed. In one study by Wennen in 1969 in The Hague, Netherlands, even babies from upper levels of the economy experienced an infant mortality of seventy per thousand, a five-hundred percent increase over the mortality in the lower income breast-fed babies. In Derby, England, according to the report of Harworth in 1905, infant mortality was seven percent among breast-fed babies and almost twenty percent among totally bottle-fed babies. These statistics have, of course, been improved with the recognition of bacteriological problems inherent in the use of cow's milk. The mortality rate has gone down precipitously with the advent of more sanitary methods. But the *morbidity* (the percentage of ill babies for one reason or another) has probably not decreased at all as we will see later.

With the advent of more canning methods, the invention of vulcanized rubber which made the artificial nipple more practical, and the introduction of condensed milk by the Nestle Company in 1866, some of the previous conditions due to bad hygiene were definitely improved. Because of these modern advances at the turn of the century and the fascination with science both in Europe and the United States, welfare agencies (and doctors) tended to promote bottle feeding as scientific and desirable. With "Modern Science" there was a rush away from "the most perfectly made solution in the world." Billions of dollars in this rich resource were thrown away, and a tremendous amount of sickness and death was caused by this great "scientific advance."

This retreat from reason and knowledge was described by William Woody, "At birth, processes are at work which are designed to enable a baby to draw its sustenance from its mother's breast; both mother and baby are physiologically prepared for this transformation. The stages of maternal lactation, the behavior of the nursling, and the nature of the required maternal responses to the baby's demands were once common knowledge."

This "common knowledge" has been almost abandoned. When I took my pediatric training in medical school in 1957, very little attention was given to breast feeding, and a great deal of time was utilized learning complicated and impractical formulas for making up a "scientific" baby mixture out of dried cow milk. Disease was all around us on the pediatric ward of this modern hospital, yet none of us realized that by promoting baby "formula," we were probably a large contributor to the misery seen around us. Jelliffee & Jelliffee have summarized eloquently in their classic work *Human Milk in the Modern World* the reasons for the dramatic drop in breast feeding from one hundred percent at the turn of the century, to thirty-eight percent in 1946, to twenty-one percent in 1956, and to a low of eighteen percent in 1966:

"The decline in breast feeding in western industrialized countries in recent decades has been due to the same forces as earlier in the Industrial Revolution, reinforced by some newer factors. For example, various feminist movements developed at the beginning of the present century, initially involved the socially well-to-do. These included the suffragette movement and earlier family planning associations with new methods of birth control. All tended to emphasize the need for a woman to strive for further economic, political, and sexual equality with men, and to endorse this by encouraging more emancipated roles, especially working outside the home. As with cigarette smoking, bobbing the hair, and the contraceptive diaphragm, the feeding bottle was also used by the "flapper" of the 1920's as a symbol of such liberation and freedom. The rise of bottle feeding also meant that the dual role of the female breast veered more to their sexual-esthetic function, with a turn to increased cultural emphasis to breast feed only in privacy. Also more recently, the western cult of ultra cleanliness, sponsored by commercially inspired anxieties about real or imaginary body odors, and the general visual and actual avoidance of human secretions, including urine, tears, sweat, nasal mucous, etc., can make breast milk as messy and even an unclean bodily discharge... which can be 'noisome to one's clothes'."[11]

In "The Cultural Warping of Childbirth," Haire (1973) reviewed the various aspects of western culture which make it often difficult for the modern mother to produce and secrete milk for her baby. These factors included:[12]

Ambivalent prenatal counselling.
Requiring all mothers to give birth in hospitals.
Elective induction of labor.

Separating the mother from familial support during labor and birth.

Withholding food and drink from normal unmedicated women in labor.

Overdependence on medication for relief of pain.

Moving normal mother to a delivery room for birth.

Delaying birth until physician arrives.

Requiring mother to assume lithotomy position.

Routine use of forceps and / or episiotomy.

Separating the mother from her newborn infant.

Use of stilbestrol for suppression of lactation.

Delaying first breast feeding.

Offering water and formula to the breast-fed newborn. Restricting newborn infants to a 4-hour schedule (and withholding night-time feedings.)

Preventing early father-child contact.

Assigning nursing personnel to mother or babies (rather than to mother-baby couples).

To the above list should be added:

Severely restricting weight gain in the prospective mother.

Cigarette smoking during pregnancy.

The use of drugs during pregnancy, including alcohol.

Berg has illustrated rather dramatically the economic impact of bottle feeding substitutes for breast feeding. He has calculated that if only one-fifth of the mothers in an urban area of a poor country do not breast feed, there is a direct loss of $365,000,000 per year. This figure must be doubled, at least, because this loss of milk must be matched by a similar expense in purchasing cow milk substitutes. Then this figure must be doubled again to pay for all of the disease and loss of brain power caused by the bottle substitution for breast milk. Everyone is losing except the manufacturers of pasteurized cow milk formula.

Reporting on the situation in Nigeria, 1969, Wennen commented:

"For the last ten years a new disease has been appearing in many developing countries; it threatens the lives of children in the first year of their existence; namely, unnecessary artificial feeding. More and more mothers start buying powdered milk for their infants even when breast milk is abundant. Incessant commercial propaganda has convinced them that 'this is good for my baby:' also the example of the 'elite mother, the fashion leader,' babies are healthy and strong . . . the result is a vicious circle of diarrhea—malnutrition, summarized in the words 'bottle disease.' "*

The blatant promotion of infant formula around the world has begun to meet with some resistance and counterattack by concerned nutritionists. An over-zealous group calling itself "Third World Working Group" produced a pamphlet on infant formula with the title *Nestlé Kills Babies.*

Nestlé counterattacked by suing the group for libel. As it turned out, this suit was eventually won by Nestle, but it was a rather empty victory. The judge decided that the term "Nestlé Kills Babies" was indeed defamatory, but he said, *the verdict was not an acquittal of Nestle,* and he instructed that Nestlé "reconsider its advertising policies to avoid being accused of immoral conduct" and to change its marketing procedures "if it does not want its product to become lethally dangerous." Toward the end of the trial Nestle withdrew three of its four libel charges. They admitted they had used nurses to promote their formula among mothers and had used questionable practices in marketing their formula.

Nestlé, because of the political pressure, promised to go straight. But according to the National Women's Health

* "Our meddling intellect mis-shapes the beauteous form of things."—Wordsworth.

Network,* they haven't done so. The National Women's Health Network continues to boycott Nestlé's baby formula, Taster's Choice coffee and other Nestlé products. Other junk food producers, quick to exploit the movement against infant formulas, are pushing sweetened condensed milk as an alternative, which may be worse. It is high in sugar and low in everything else.

The Protein Advisory Group of the United Nations has been attempting for a number of years to stop some of the unethical disastrous practices of the baby food industry with no real success. At a meeting in 19 7 3, a tentative code of practice was drafted, but it has not been followed by the food industry. That code read in part as follows:

> "No claim shall be made in an advertisement implying that any food, including infant formula, is equivalent or superior to mother's milk, nor shall statements be made in advertisements which would, directly or indirectly, encourage mothers not to breast feed their infants. No advertisement shall state or imply that the product advertised had medical or other professional support."

Mead Johnson stretches and bends this code to the limit in their advertising to doctors. They continue their vain attempt to imitate mother's milk with their "improved formulation" of Enfamil. Their concoction of 55% coconut and 45% soy oil has, they say, a fatty acid level "within the range of breast milk values" and is "nutritionally unsurpassed."

A fatty acid called linolinic acid is extremely important in human nutrition, perhaps more important than some of the vitamins. The immature physiology of a baby may not be able to transform the fatty acid linoleic to the essential linolinic acid. But nature has protected the human baby, and none other, from this deficiency. Human milk is the only known animal source of this important vitamin-like substance.

---

* They are very female chauvinistic, but they do a lot of good. Their address is: 2 24 Seventh St., SE, Washington, D.C. 2 0003.

What Mead doesn't tell the doctors in their advertising is that coconut oil is unfit for babies or adults and that the vital linolinic acid of mother's milk is totally absent from their "improved formulation." And worse, the trans fatty acids in their product may block the baby from making any of this vital nutrient. So the next time you see some hyperactive kid climbing the walls, ask the mother if he was bottle-fed.

Milk From Unusual Places

There are some really strange things going on in the breast milk world. Women who have adopted babies *and have never been pregnant* have learned to produce perfectly normal milk. A study in 1981[13] reviewed "induced lactation" in two hundred forty adoptive mothers.

Half of these women through strong mental attitude (oxytocin production) and nipple stimulation (prolactin production) were able to produce milk even before the baby was obtained! Women who had lactated before from a pregnancy were three times as likely to succeed at induced lactation, also called adoptive nursing. Supplemental feeding was gradually decreased as breast milk increased in supply. None of the infants became dehydrated or failed to gain weight.

The editor of the journal in which this report appeared felt constrained to refute the basic premise of the article. He said, "The title of this report suggests that nonpuerperal (not pregnant) adoptive mothers were somehow able to secrete milk for their infants... true lactation does not occur under circumstances described here ...Attempts to nourish a baby by a nonpuerperal mother cannot provide a mother's milk...: Ed."*

You were amazed to find that non-pregnant women can nurse? Wait until you read this next part.**

---

* Ed, you're dead wrong.
** You're not going to believe it.

There's an herb grown in Guatemala and the surrounding countries called "ixbut," pronounced "iss' boot."[14] This herb is said to be a powerful galactagogue.* A report in "Flora of Guatemala" states that ixbut will double the quantity of milk from cows and that a broth of it will greatly increase milk flow in lactating mothers. It is also claimed that ixbut will cause milk production in non-pregnant women. Countless tales are heard in Guatemala about the wondrous powers of ixbut. It is claimed that aged grandmothers and even great-grandmothers, through the magic of ixbut, can nurse babies through their withered breasts!

Bertha Garcia, a teacher with a nutritional institute in Guatemala, authenticated one case.[15] While on a dietary survey, she met a forty-five year old Indian woman who was nursing a small fourteen-month old baby. The mother of the baby, her sister, had died in childbirth. They were too poor to buy milk for the baby, so the aunt, who had not nursed a baby in twenty-five years, took it upon herself to nurse the baby. She took ixbut tea for several months and nursed successfully. Garcia, skeptical about her claim, asked to see her breasts. There was no doubt that she was lactating normally.

But here's the real show-stopper as reported by Rosengarten: [16]

> "An even more curious incident involving ixbut was reported in a Guatemalan newspaper in November, 1952: During the late 1890's, a Guatemalan physician, Dr. Pedro Molina, was at his home near Flores, Peten. One afternoon, he received a message that he was urgently needed by a woman in labor. By the time he arrived at the isolated, humble, native hut, he managed to save the life of the baby girl, but the mother died. Dr. Molina thereupon asked the feeble great-grandfather, who appeared to be at least ninety years old, what woman was going to nurse the infant. This venerable progenitor replied that no woman was around, but no woman was in fact needed since he himself

---

* Black's Medical Dictionary: "Galactagogues are drugs which increase the flow of milk in nursing women."

would be the wet nurse; he was going to drink a tea of the medicinal herbixbut which would enable him to provide milk for his new greatgranddaughter. The physician objected and reluctantly departed. Six days later, Dr. Molina returned to check on the condition of the baby; he found the old man boiling ixbut leaves in a pot of water; for five days he had been dr~nking the infusion, but he complained that his swollen breasts hurt him when the infant suckled. The physician examined the great-grandfather's breasts which indeed were enlarged like the teats of a perfect wet nurse and were exuding a milky juice that tasted like mother's milk. The baby was thriving."*

Before you laugh that story off you should know that bulls have been induced to lactate by hormonal manipulation. Professor W.E. Peterson reported[17] that bulls and steers have been made to produce milk in small amounts that was normal in character.

What To Do

Concerning the breast milk/cow milk formula controversy, much can be done to help the United States (and the world) get back to basic breast feeding.

We must encourage medical schools to increase the time allowed for teaching the importance of breast feeding infants. The book by Jelliffee entitled Human Milk and the Modern World should become a basic textbook in every medical school in the United States. Nurses and other paramedical personnel need, of course, to receive similar education.

Legislators and other leaders in the community need to be apprised of the situation as it exists today. I would recommend that copies of this book be given to people in positions of influence. For the professional, I would again recommend HumanMilkand theModern World byJelliffee & Jelliffee.

As far as educating the general public is concerned, the LaLeche League is the single best way to get the infor-

---

* I'm not sure I believe it, either.

mation to the general public. This is a very cooperative and enthusiastic organization that will help you in any way that they possibly can to help educate the people in your community as to the importance of breast feeding.

Pressure must be put on the various baby formula companies to discourage them from their unethical and counter-productive practices. These companies are very sensitive to criticism, especially when it is public.

Every effort should be made to keep the commercial formula companies from unduly influencing school children as to the importance of natural feeding. The commercial milk companies do an excellent job with beautiful, expensive brochures and scientific material, to present their side to the school children. To put it mildly, the National Dairy Council has been extremely successful in this regard.

Jack Mathis, President of Mathis Dairy, Atlanta, Georgia, remarked in a talk to the National Health Federation, that his dairy has for a number of years routinely taken colostrum from the cow and frozen it so as to have it handy in case of illness in a calf. He found that when the calf becomes ill and is fed colostrum it will almost always rapidly improve. Without the colostrum the calf will often die.

There is no reason why this same principle cannot apply in human medicine. Breast banks were not uncommon in earlier decades of this century. We need to go back and investigate these banks and put them in use wherever practicable.

REFERENCES

1. Sheehan & Davis, 1968.

2. Klagsbrun, et al, J. Surg. Res., 26, 417-422 (1979).

3. Sinclair & Crawford, 1973.

4. Pediatrics, Volume 64, Nr. 4, pp. 550.

5. Johnson & Salisbury, 1975.

6. Human Milk in the Modern World, Oxford University Press, 1978.

7. New Zealand Med. Journal, Vol. 76, #482, 1972, pp. 28-31.

8. Hollen, Journal Ped. Env. Child. Health, 20, 288, 1976.

9. Grulee, 1934.

10. Jelliffee & Jelliffee, 1975-1976.

11. Wickes, 1953.

12. Op. cit., pp. 193.

13. Obstetrical & Gynecological Survey, Vol. 36, Nr. 11, November 1981.

14. Botanical Museum Leallets, Harvard University, Vol. 26, Nr. 9-10, pp. 277.

15. Op. cit., pp. 278.

16. Op. cit., pp. 278.

17. Discussion at the annual Convention of the Milk Industry Foundation, Atlantic City, New Jersey, October 18, 1950.

Chapter X

"THIS GREASY COUNTERFEIT"

"Butter and eggs are the innocent victims of the... anti-cholesterol establishment which attempts to replace proven foods
with untried substitutes."[1]
Kurt A. Oster, M.D.

In 1886 the first great impassioned controversy in
the Congress developed involving a pure food issue. This
issue was over oleomargarine and whether it should
have "equal protection" with butter. A bill was introduced in Congress to place a tax on oleomargarine.
Never before in the history of the Congress had there
been such a hot and emotional debate over food. Representative William Hatch of Missouri termed the controversy the "most remarkable elementary contest that has
been on this floor for many years."

The issue excited a great public interest. In the
words of Representative Warner Miller of New York, it
would be "a new species of legislation, or largely so, in
this country and into our system." A South Carolina senator termed it "the most flagrant, unblushing disregard of
the principles of the constitution that has ever been introduced into the Congress."

Emperor Napolean III had personally promoted the
quest to find a substitute for butter which would be less
expensive and of better keeping qualities. A French food
chemist by the name of Hippolyte Mege-Mouriez* patented his invention of oleomargarine in 1869. He had
done his research on the royal farms of Napoleon III at
Vincennes. Mege began to manufacture his "beurre
economique" in Paris just after the outbreak of the
Franco-Prussian War.**

---

* We'll just call him Mege.
** Ironically, no French chef who takes pride in his sauté would ever use
    margarine.

In 1873 the United States Dairy Company of New York City acquired the Mege patent and began producing oleomargarine. Many Americans at this time, some one hundred-eighty in all, applied for similar artificial butter patents.

Dairymen immediately began to react to this competition and began to have laws passed to regulate the sale of oleomargarine. In 1884 New York actually passed a law banning oleomargarine completely, but this was declared unconstitutional by the New York Supreme Court.

Mege's system of production of margarine was bizarre. He used chopped up stomachs of cattle, finely chopped udders of cows or hogs or ewes, added carbonated soda, coloring matter, and salt to create this new food, called oleomargarine. As James Harvey Young stated, "What lured them, the Chicago Meat Packers, was a desire to put to profitable use everything but the pig's squeal."[2] The packers used "neutral" pork fat by using a new deodorizing process. The pork fat was mixed with beef fat and then pressed through a cloth to separate the oleo oil. This was sometimes mixed with milk or cream to make a high grade of oleo. They called the mixture "Butterine." The manufacturers preferred this name to oleomargarine. There were many variations to this technique, depending on the manufacturers. They were careful to package the product in tubs shaped just like those traditionally used for butter.

This "Butterine" was aggressively marketed and was often fraudently sold at the retail level as butter. As the imitation butter bit deeper into the natural butter market, dairymen reacted even more strongly and set up a convention to pass national laws against the misrepresentation of "Butterine" and oleomargarine. From this convention a bill was formulated and was presented to the Congress of the United States in 1886. It quickly passed the House, and after some modification by the Senate, it was signed into law by President Grover Cleveland.

Senator Bob LaFollette, never at a loss for words, had this to say, "Ingenuity, striking hands with cunning trickery, compounds a substance to counterfeit an article of food. It is made to look like something it is not; to taste and smell like something it is not; to sell like something it is not; and so deceive the purchaser. This monstrous product of greed and hypocrisy makes its way into the home and on the table of every consumer. Here is a villainous device for making money lawlessly, subtly, eating the heart out of an industry which is to the government what blood is to the body."

The fight in Congress made it clear that this was not a nutritional issue at that time but an economic one. As pointed out by Young, one man in a single factory could make more margarine than all of the butter that all of New York's farmers could produce put together.

A Chicago representative claimed that the bill to tax oleomargarine was a blatant attempt "to revive the drooping dairy interests." The "drooping dairy interests" had indeed brought the bill about. Farming was greatly depressed, and the dairy industry was justifiably concerned about the impact of this new butter substitute, oleomargarine.

The defenders of oleomargarine pointed out that new inventions often cause the demise of the old. They claimed that this was a great invention of modern science and should not be obstructed because of dairy interests. They even went so far as to claim that oleomargarine was better than butter.* Dr. Charles F. Chandler, a medical professor from Columbia College of Medicine, even went so far as to testify that margarine *was* butter made by a safe new process. Replying to this, Senator Palmer called oleo the "monumental fraud of the 19th century."

With remarkable prescience which has only begun to be appreciated today, D.E. Salmon, Chief of Bureau of Animal Industry, said that an invention like oleomargarine "which introduces a radical change to the manufacture of an article of food which goes on the table of every

---

*Doctors are now telling their patients the same thing.

family in the land *might produce an unexpected and remarkable effect on the public health."* (Emphasis added.)

Salmon had sounded a very wise and justified word
of caution, but it added to the hysteria among the defenders of butter. Witnesses testifying before the House
Committee asserted, "Dead horses, dead cows, and even
dead dogs, when they had been shot for hydrophobia,
and other carcasses of the city were... taken to a rendering establishment... where the great bulk of these things
were made into 'pure' oleo oil." Dr. Thomas Taylor of the
Department of Agriculture suggested that margarine factories might be the destination for drowned sheep and
for hogs dead from cholera and from a diet of distillery
swill. A North Carolina Congressman said that margarine
was the sort of carrion that only jackals and turkey buz-
zards reveled in.

A spokesman for the leading margarine* manufacturers replied that only fresh fat was used in their product. The friends of butter remained skeptical.

But many times over it was shown during the house
reports by members of the Congress that strong acids and
alkalies were being used to deodorize stale and noxious
fats to make "bastard butter."

Representative Grout, "Who will say that the things
we eat are not, like Caesar's wife, to be above suspicion?"
The oleo manufacturers defended themselves against
these charges and denied using most of the fifty dangerous ingredients that had been cited in testimony.

Another serious charge leveled at the oleo makers
by the dairy interests was that bacteria, parasites, spores,
mold, hair, bristles, and portions of worms were to be
found in the oleo. This "cheap, nasty grease" could be fatal, according to a North Carolina representative who

---

* It should be pronounced as in Margaret, a hard "G" as the word comes
  from the Greek margarites meaning "pearl-like". Forget it.

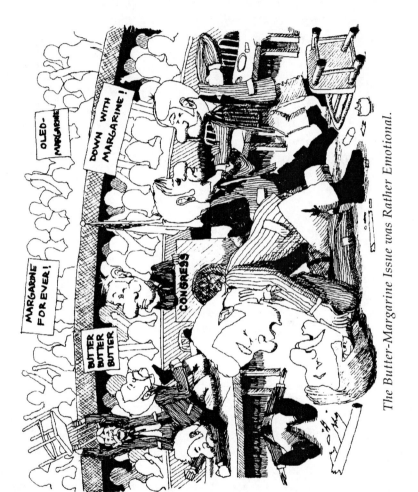

The Butter-Margarine Issue was Rather Emotional.

said that many of those who ate it might have a coroner's verdict of "died of bogus butter." Animal fat, countered the defenders of oleo, did not contain germs and worms which were only found in the muscle of animals. Therefore, they said, the charges were ridiculous.

The oleo manufacturers asserted that their product was equal to the best butter and was in fact perhaps superior. They noted that the dairymen were not always clean in their habits or above reproach, that butter was sometimes adulterated with beets, carrots, and potatoes. That, in fact, dairies often bought oleo oil to supplement their cream. While condemning the oleo manufacturers for coloring their product, they asserted butter makers resorted to dyes to color their own product.

In desperation the dairy industry introduced legislation to tax oleo out of existence. After a very emotional debate, a law was passed in 1886 which taxed oleomargarine to remove its economic advantage over butter. Another fiery debate took place in 1948 (See Appendix V), but in 1950 the tax on margarine was removed. It took 64 years.

Although motivated by profit just as much as the oleo manufacturers, subsequent research has proven the dairy interests to be correct in many of their accusations concerning the nutritional shortcomings of oleo.

Dr. T.W. Gullickson, Professor of Dairy Chemistry, University of Minnesota, proved the nutritional superiority of butterfat over vegetable oils, which are the main ingredients of the vegetable margarines. Gullickson used skim milk and combined it with lard, tallow, coconut oil, corn oil, cottonseed oil or soybean oil in place of the cream and fed it to calves. The vegetable oil substitutes were mixed with skim milk in an attempt to imitate the 3.5 percent butterfat of milk. As often happens in research, they proved something entirely different from their original objective. They had set out to find a cheaper way to raise calves for veal production. What they found was that calves will only grow on God's own natural milk, and when fed vegetable oil substitutes instead of the cream, they sicken and die.

On the corn oil mix three out of eight died within one hundred-seventy days, some as soon as thirty-three days. On cottonseed oil three out of four died within one hundred-twenty-six days. Pick your favorite vegetable oil —the result was the same. The survivors quickly recovered when switched to whole raw milk. If vegetable oil products are so devastating to the health of calves, do you think maybe they are bad for you, too?

The American Medical Association took cognizance of these significant findings, "...the consuming public has a right to demand that the practice of clearly distinguishing between margarine and butter, so that every one can recognize them, be continued."

Professor T.H. Frandsen, Department of Dairy Industry, Massachusetts State College, was even more adamant,[3] "Butter and margarine should be advertised and sold for exactly what they are. There should be no attempt to deceive or pawn off margarine for butter ..."

The current practice, encouraged by doctors and the American Heart Association, of increasing the consumption of vegetable oils in the diet is a nutritional disaster. Unsaturated fatty acids are needed only in small amounts in the diet. They are in adequate supply in vegetables, nuts, and meat. It would be difficult, even in the average American diet, not to get adequate amounts of unsaturated fats.

Unsaturated fats found in vegetable oils increase the production of "free radicals," which are by-products of cellular chemistry. They are like tiny hand grenades that devastate body tissues, leading to degeneration and early aging. These little free radical killers lead to hardening of the arteries and cancer.

In fact, the major cause of aging is probably "free

radical" formation.* Free radicals are atoms with an electrical charge on them. NACL is a balanced compound.
Take away the Na (sodium) and you have a free radical
of chlorine, a Cl⁻. These are the terrorists in your body
that probably cause hardening of the arteries, leading to
strokes and heart attacks.

The reason the oils are called "polyunsaturated" is
because they have many electrons like the Cl⁻, in their
structure. They look like this: $c = c—c = c—c—c =$. When
they are oxidized in the body, they form many free radicals which can attack your blood vessels.**

Dr. Denham Harman, an authority on free radical
chemistry and physiology, has stated that a reduction in
these harmful reactions through dietary changes and/or
the addition of protective elements in the diet would
have a drastic effect. "This approach offers the prospect
of an increase in the average life expectancy to beyond 85
years and a significant increase in the number of people
who will live to well beyond 100 years."

Modern medicine, using a chemical approach, has
failed to achieve this. The mean life span has remained
virtually constant at 70 years since the mid-1950's. This
life expectancy may well decrease in the future if we continue to be seduced by the false nutritional propaganda
of the vegetable oil producers.

Harman studied the effect of various fats and oils on
mice. He found that rats fed lard lived 9.2% longer than

---

* A "free radical" is not an American communist. You need to
understand what a free radical is in order to understand why you
should use lard or butter for cooking rather than the polyunsaturated
oils.

** Smog also contains many free radicals. That's one good argument for
atomic power.

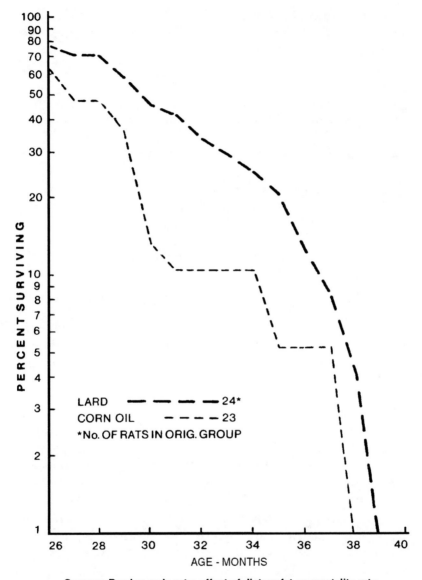

Sprague-Dawley male rats: effect of dietary fat on mortality rate.

From *The Journal of the American Geriatrics Society,* Vol XVII, Aug. 1969, #8, p. 727.

rats fed a polyunsaturate.* In humans that translates to almost 7 years off your life if you have been suckered into television nutrition and American Heart Association anticholesterol propaganda.

If the unsaturated oil and lard are pushed to 20% of the total diet (well within the range of human consumption), the life span of the rats consuming the unsaturated oil was 17% less than those fed lard. Assuming a 70-year life span of man, this translates to almost 12 years less life for the oil consumers as compared to lard users.

Research at the University of Georgia on various fats helped to exonerate the fat of red meat.[5] They found that adding stearate fat (from animals) to the diet of rats lowered cholesterol levels. Vegetable fats had no effect. The stearate also lowered blood pressure.**

Atherosclerosis isn't the only disease the polyunsaturated oils can give you. Cancer can be induced in experimental animals with corn oil.[6] Hypertension will occur in rats and chickens by feeding unsaturated oils whereas animal fats (lard, milk, butter) do not cause high blood pressure. Amyloidosis, a disease of protein degeneration, can also be induced by polyunsaturates.[7]

The trans fatty acids of margarine, a solid form of vegetable oil, may even change the very function of some cells.[8] One country, alarmed at the dramatic increase in unsaturated fatty acid and resaturated fatty acid consumption, has strictly limited their content in foods such as margarine. Our government remains unconcerned.[9]

Rosenfield, in the September issue of Science '81, said, "Wouldn't it be ironic... if, having switched to polyunsaturates in order to prolong our lives by preventing atherosclerosis and heart attacks, we were instead

---

* He used safflower oil. Corn oil is even worse.
** But these studies will have to be repeated. They were financed by the National Dairy Council and the National Live Stock and Meat Board.

shortening our lives by prematurely aging our cells and perhaps even creating additional cancer risks?"

A spokesman for the London Coronary Prevention Group, Dr. Keith Ball,[10] takes the position that fat is fat. Ball said, "It is not always appreciated that butter is also, in effect, an hydrogenated product..."

What he does not tell us is that the fatty acids made by the cow are very different from those made in the margarine plant by man. The "cis" transfiguration of the fatty acids in butter look like this:

. They are entirely digestible. The "trans" form, made at the margarine plant by bombarding a vegetable oil with hydrogen and nickel, looks like this:

. It was not intended by nature to be used as food and, in fact, rarely occurs in nature.

Ball gives a hard pitch for margarine and a low saturated fat diet, "The fat switch from butter and other saturated fats to polyunsaturated oils and margarine has a sound nutritional basis." He laments the fact that low fat milk is not readily available in England because "...only excess fat in milk is considered harmful." (See effects of low fat milk on health, Chapter m.)

Ball defends his position on the saturated/unsaturated fat issue,[11] "...there is complete agreement by all twenty international committees... that there should be a reduction of saturated fat in countries with high coronary mortality rates."

Among this impressive group of twenty is the Royal College of Physicians, the British Cardiac Society, and Ball's organization, the Coronary Prevention Group, London. This is an impressive array of committees, but remember the definition of a camel: A greyhound designed by a committee. The facts simply don't substantiate their encouragement of unsaturated fat consumption in place of saturated fat, butter, and meat.

Man has been eating meat and fat for thousands of years, but hardening of the arteries is a new disease. My father, practicing medicine in Georgia fifty years ago, rarely saw a heart attack. Heart attacks have only become common since the advent of homogenized pasteurized milk, oleomargarine, and the increased consumption of polyunsaturated vegetable oils.

A quick tour through the supermarkets will show you that in spite of these disturbing findings on the deleterious effects of oleomargarine it is winning the battle for the dinner table every year.* The butter section seems to get smaller and the oleo section larger. A study of southern households reported in the Journal of the American Dietetic Association (July, 1980) revealed that margarine was purchased twelve times more often than butter. Even farm families use margarine primarily. One University of Georgia coed with whom we are acquainted had never tasted butter until she visited the home of a friend in Atlanta. She was from a small south Georgia farm town and grew up around cows!

As margarine is a water and oil mixture, these elements must be mechanically forced together. They are naturally unwilling partners. This is basically a homogenization process, and some of the same nutritional problems arise as we have with homogenized milk. There is no xanthine oxidase (xo) in margarine. But instead of abnormally small natural animal fat particles slipping into the blood stream as in homogenized milk, we now have abnormally small unnatural vegetable oil such as corn, cottonseed, and coconut oils going into the blood stream through lymphatic channels.

"So what?" you say. The experts tell me margarine is better for me—no cholesterol, no animal fat to harden my arteries.

---

*By 1982 margarine had captured 72% of the buttermarket.

These oils are as refined as the gasoline in your car. In the refinery they are treated with a caustic soda solution which removes the lecithin, an essential nutrient.* Then the oil is steam-cleaned under a vacuum at tremendous temperature. This second step should destroy any remaining food value in the oil, but, just in case, the oil is then bleached at a high temperature to remove any color.

The liquid oil is then chemically treated by being bombarded with hydrogen under pressure in the presence of the metal nickel. This "hydrogenation" process is what makes the oil look like real butter. But now it's no longer a "polyunsaturate" which is supposed to be so good for you.

The remaining step in the manufacture of plastic butter is to steam clean it *again* at high temperatures to deodorize it. Then the preservatives and color are added, and it is ready for your table.

The liquid part of margarine, which is the second largest component, is usually *re-pasteurized*, that is reheated, skim milk. So the butter substitute on your toast has been steam-cleaned or superheated at least *four times.*

In England butter is rapidly disappearing. It costs twice as much as margarine, and the average English consumer, not aware of the nutritional problems with margarine, is unwilling to pay the price.** The North European Dairy Journal comments, "...it will only be a few years before the English dairy industry will be in great need of their own consumers in order to sell their product." This is a worldwide trend. Margarine has definitely taken over.

Both World Wars, with their shortage of fat, stimulated the use of margarine. Cheap, imported coconut oil became a dominant factor in margarine, and the butter interests began attacking this "coconut cow."[12] The imported coconut oil was seen as an economic threat to the farmer. Little did

---

* As with most refined products, they throw it back in later.
** He may pay the price later in poor health.

they know that it would also prove to be a threat to the health of the consumer as well. (See Chapter VIII.)

Southern farmers jumped into the fray on the side of margarine. You can't eat cotton, but the cotton has a seed, and the seed contains oil. It is even more indigestible than our interloper from the soap factory coconut oil, but at least it's home-grown. Southerners grumbled that northern states discriminated against them by their state laws,[13] and in retaliation some southern states taxed margarine made from imported coconut oil.

By the end of World War II the margarines were almost pure vegetable oil. Eliminating the more expensive animal fat* greatly reduced cost. This had a devastating effect on the butter industry which could not hope to compete on a price basis. The average cost of oleomargarine in 1930 was twenty cents a pound. The average cost of the all vegetable margarine in 1941, eleven years later, was only seventeen cents per pound.

To make matters worse for the butter industry, their production costs after the war increased dramatically. By 1947, butter was one dollar a pound.

But the final battle in the butter/margarine war was not fought in the Congress or at the supermarket. The victory was handed to the margarine manufacturers by American medicine. The animal fat—cholesterol paradigm, which states that they cause hardening of the arteries, put the checkmate on the butter knights. Nothing remains but a mopping up operation.** Even India is giving up its traditional ghee, made from buffalo milk fat, for vanaspati —a vegetable oil substitute.

---

* Which eliminated the need for the oleo part of the word, oleomargarine.

** By 1970, Americans were consuming ten pounds of margarine per person per year. That doesn't leave much room for butter.

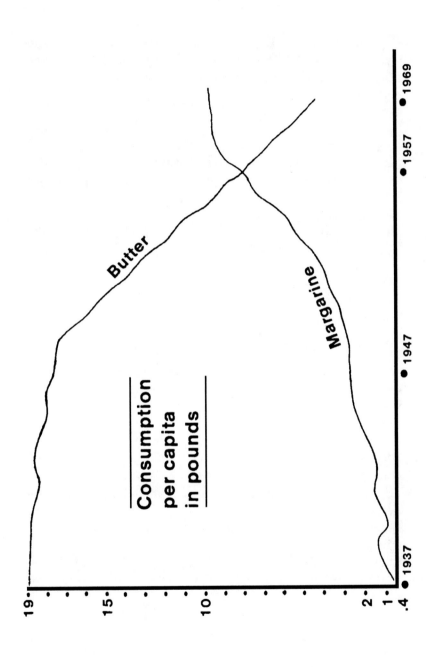

Consumption
per capita
in pounds

Butter

Margarine

19
15
10
2
1
.4

1937 1947 1957 1969

Animal fat consumption has not increased in the past sixty years. The increase in heart attacks has paralleled the increased consumption of margarine, homogenized milk, and other processed foods.

"Okay, so I might get a heart attack from eating margarine. But the American Cancer Society, the National Cancer Institute, and the Senate Committee on Nutrition and Human Needs all say that animal fat, such as butter, may give me cancer of the colon. Certainly *they* couldn't all be wrong."*

The Senate Committee mentioned above published a report entitled *Dietary Goals for the United States*.[14] The committee came down hard on saturated fat relating it to ". . . six of the ten leading causes of death. . ." Down with saturated and up with unsaturated fat, they recommended. Everyone agreed.** Thence began the rush to the sea— coconut, cottonseed, corn, palm, and soybean oils; skim milk; "whitener"; eggbeaters. What did we find when we got there? More atherosclerosis, not less.

A group of bright graduate students at the University of Maryland Department of Chemistry and Dairy Science scratched their heads and wondered if maybe these prestigious societies, institutes, and select committees were going in the wrong direction.[15] Why did the situation get worse instead of better when the diet was changed from animal fat to vegetable fat?

The facts are quite different from what is generally believed. The percentage of *animal* fat in the diet has steadily *decreased* over the past sixty years. The percentage of *vegetable* fat in the diet has increased markedly in this same period, about 400%. The proportion of animal fat in the American diet dropped from 83% in 1910 to 62% in 1972.

---

* Yes, they could.
** Including me, at the time.

The Maryland investigators restudied the Senate committee's sources of information and found that their conclusions implicating animal fat in cancer were the result of errors in arithmetic! The dramatic increase in fat consumption was not from animal fat as reported by the Senate Committee but a 90% increase in *vegetable oils* and *margarine consumption.*

There is a great deal of misunderstanding, even among scientists, about which fats are saturated and which are not. How many people realize that coconut oil, which is used extensively in candy, baby formula, baked goods, fake milk, and many other junk foods, is *over twice* as saturated as pork fat?[16] Beef fat is only 48% saturated, pork fat 40% saturated, but coconut oil is 95% saturated. In fact, since 1929, more saturated fat in the diet has come from vegetable fat than from beef. Yet Wynder, in 1975, editorialized[17] that beef was "...the major source of saturated fat in the adult population of the United States."

The experts on the Senate Select Committee claim that countries with a high animal fat intake have higher rates of colon and breast cancer. This is simply not true. In fact, the opposite appears more likely.

Take Finland and the Netherlands for example.[18] Their per capita daily *animal* fat consumption is the same. But the Dutch consume *four times* as much vegetable fat as the Finns, and they have *twice* the rate of colon and breast cancer. Many other examples could be cited.[19]

Eng and co-workers at the University of Maryland did a statistical analysis of the same USDA data relied on by the Senate Committee. They found a *"strong significant positive correlation* with ...vegetable fat, and *an essentially strong negative correlation* ...with animal fat to total cancer deaths (and) breast and colon cancer incidence."

In plain language, you are more likely to get cancer from vegetable fat, such as margarine, than you are from animal fat such as butter. "Negative correlation" means that despite what the experts said, butter and other animal fats may be *protective* from cancer!

Promoters of the animal fat theory of cancer causation don't like to be reminded that Tannenbaum, in his
original work thirty-five years ago on dietary fat and
cancer, used hydrogenated cottonseed oil and soybean
oil, not animal fat.

The major factor causing vegetable fats to be carcinogenic is probably the hydrogenation process which changes
the unsaturated fatty acids to the trans form. We described
this on page 179. The trans fatty acids accumulate in the
blood cells causing them to explode.[20]. They probably accumulate in most organs of the body and they cause swelling
of liver cells.[21]. Margarine and vegetable shortenings may
contain as much as 47% and 58% respectively of trans fatty
acids. Think about *that* the next time you butter your toast
with "nature's own" corn oil margarine.

Not that some unsaturated fatty acids in their unal-
tered state aren't important. There's a whole new class of
vitamin-like substances called the "F complex." It includes unpronounceable things like eicosapentonoic acid
and docohexanoic acid. But you don't get these from the
oils and margarine sold in your local supermarket. Find a
good nutritionist and discuss it with him. It's important.

Why did the McGovern Committee ignore the scientific literature incriminating vegetable fats in atherosclerosis? Extensive studies[22] with monkeys fed vegetable
oils proved beyond a doubt that peanut oil, coconut oil,
and other vegetable fats cause severe hardening of the arteries. With the current fixation on cholesterol in the nutritional establishment, it is important to note that on
peanut oil the serum cholesterol remained low. The peanut oil may kill you, but you can die with a normal cholesterol.*

Dr. Elspeth B. Smith, Department of Pathology, University of Aberdeen, Scotland, remarked on this extremely important vegetable oil research in a letter to the British

---

*Jimmy Carter is not going to like this.

Journal, Lancet:[23] "Inexplicably, this work is totally ignored by advocates of dietary change although it emanates from a leading... laboratory in Chicago, and not from a crank in an obscure institute.* It is ignored both at the clinical level, *and by the many committees set up to make dietary recommendations...*" (Emphasis added.)

By implication, Smith says, the polyunsaturates promoters support the following formulas:

Animal fat= butter = saturated fat= BAD
Polyunsaturated= vegetable= GOOD**

Smith suggests that these misled scientists stop "... campaigning for destruction of the dairy industry which produces their milk, the cheapest source of first class protein available."

Other than the fact that margarine may kill you, what else is wrong with it? An English institution for boys ran a nutritional experiment in 1938.[24] A group of boys were fed one and three-fourths ounces of New Zealand "grass-fed butter." Another group was fed margarine. The margarine proved "worthless for growth," but the butter group grew an extra .38 inches during the experimental period. The investigators had previously done a similar test on rats. They concluded, "There is something in butter that isn't in margarine and it works on boys the same as on rats."

The food engineers seem determined to wipe out the entire dairy industry.*** Europeans are now producing margarine cheese. The price differential will be enormously in favor of fake cheese guaranteeing its popularity. It is so much like real cheese that "if a cheese made with vegetable oil was judged together with other cheese,

---

* Not that "cranks" aren't occasionally right. Some people think I'm a crank.
** Butter is only 65% saturated; coconut oil is 95%.
*** And maybe the human race.

it is doubtful whether anyone would realize that a margarine cheese was among them."[25]

Many restaurants keep their cooking oil and reheat it, adding additional oil as needed. That's a lot cheaper than starting over every day. But prolonged heating and reheating of unsaturated oil causes "polymerization" which turns the oil into shellac and varnish. Pinckney reported[26] that animals fed these oils often develop intestinal blockage.*

If you eat commercial food, it is hard to get away from these oils because they put them into practically everything as a stabilizer. "Brominated" vegetable oils are added to ice cream, soft drinks and bakery products.**

Crest Foods of Ashton, Illinois now produces vegetable fat "sour cream." It is doubly pasteurized and homogenized at least twice.*** The fats used in Crest's "sour cream" are our friends from the soap factory, coconut oil and palm kernel oil.

"Bogus butter" and its friends have won hands down. Margarine is king.

---

* The animals were often found with their little butts *stuck to the cage floor* because of varnish feces.

** No wonder everybody is constipated.

*** We've told you what homogenization does to milk and what it will do to you. As far as we know, no one has investigated what homogenization of vegetable fat does to you—should be interesting.

REFERENCES

1. Nutrition Today, November/December, 1981.

2. Bulletin History of Medicine, Nr. 53, 1979.

3. Certified Milk Magazine, December, 1944.

4. *Prolongation of Life: Role of Free Radical Reactions in Aging,* Harman, J. Am. Gen. Soc., SVII, 8, August 1969.

5. Resurreccion, Coster and Bargmann, Univ. of Georgia. (Remainder of reference missing.)

6. Gamal, et al, Cancer Res. 27:1787, 1967.

7. Cohen, N.E.J. Med. 277:522, 574, 628 (1967).

8. Fed. Proc., July 1978, pp. 2215.

9. Fredricks, Prevention Magazine, November 1981.

10. Lancet, April 22, 1980.

11. Lancet, February 2, 1980.

12. *The Story of Margarine,* Riepma, Public Affairs Press, 1970.

13. U.S.D.A., State and Federal Legislations and Decisions Relating to Oleomargarine, Washington, 1936.

14. Washington, D.C., 1977, Sen. George McGovern, Chairman.

15. *Dietary Fat and Cancer Trends, A Critique Enig.,* et al, Federation Proceedings, Vol. 37, Nr. 9, 1978.

16. Rizek, et al, J. Amer. Oil Chem. Soc., 51:244, 1974. 17. Wynder & Reddy, J. Nat'l. Cancer Inst., 54:7, 1975.

17. Carroll, Cancer Rev. 35:3374, 1975; Gregor, et al, 10:1031, 1969.

18. Enig., et al, Fed. Proc., Vol. 37, Nr. 9, July 1978, pp. 2215-2220.

19. Decker & Mertz, J. Nuts, 89:165, 1966; J. Nuts, 91:324, 1967.

20. Ibid.

21. Wiegand, Acta Med. Scan. 1959, 166 sup 351.

22. The Lancet, March 8, 1981.

23. Physical Culture Mag., July, 1939.

24. North European Dairy Journal, May 1981.

25. Pinckney, *The Cholesterol Controversy*, Sherbourne Press, L.A., 1973.

Chapter XI

UDDERLY EFFECTIVE
(Milk as Medicine)

William Osler, the most respected physician of the early 20th Century, said, "A rigid milk diet may be tried . . . this plan in conjunction with rest is most efficacious." And then he quoted Cheynes, "Milk and sweet sound blood differ in nothing but color: Milk is blood."

"The dividing line between a food and a medicine sometimes becomes almost invisible. In many diseases nothing heals the body and restores strength like milk."...

Dr. J.F. Lyman, Prof. of Agricultural Chemistry, Ohio State University, 1928.

One of the most remarkable and important discoveries in medicine, the increadible healing power of fresh raw milk, goes unnoticed by the medical profession. No one knows who first used raw milk as a therapeutic agent, probably Hippocrates, the father of medicine, who prescribed it for tuberculosis.

We pick up the story in 1929 at the Mayo Foundation, Rochester, Minnesota. Dr. J.E. Crewe reported, "While milk is widely used and recommended as an article of diet, it is seldom used by regular physicians exclusively as an agent in the treatment of disease. For fifteen years I have employed the so-called milk treatment in various diseases... *the results obtained in various types of illnesses have been so uniformly excellent that one's conception of disease and its alleviation is necessarily modified.*"[1] (Emphasis added.)

Dr. Crewe, taking a weary look at his colleagues said laconically, "The method itself is so simple that it does not greatly interest medical men."[2] And then, taking a not only weary, but a wary look at his associates said, "The fact that many diseases are treated and successful results claimed, leads almost to disrespect."

Even advanced cases of pulmonary tuberculosis improved rapidly with milk therapy. (Hippocrates told doctors hundreds of years ago that milk would greatly alleviate tuberculosis.) This was ironic in that raw milk was being blamed, incorrectly, for a great deal of the tuberculosis seen in that decade.

His report on the treatment of edema (swelling) is even more striking, "In cases in which there is marked edema, the results obtained are surprisingly marked. This is especially striking because so-called dropsy has never been treated with large quantities of fluid. With all medication withdrawn, one case lost twenty-six pounds in six days, huge edema disappearing from the abdomen and legs with great relief to the patient."

Patients with heart failure were taken off medications, including digitalis (Lanoxin), and "responded splendidly." Especially satisfactory, Crewe reported, was the treatment of high blood pressure with the milk diet: "High blood pressure patients respond splendidly and the results in most instances are quite lasting."

Perhaps the most startling treatment, and one that goes counter to present-day thinking, was obesity. Raw milk, with all that fat, for the treatment of obesity? Dr. Crewe: "One patient reduced from 325 pounds to 284 pounds in two weeks, on four quarts of milk a day while her blood pressure was reduced from 220 to 170."

Although Dr. Crewe's experiments were on the feeding of *raw milk* for disease, the key is not *milk*, but *raw*. The same results might be obtained, as Crewe implies, by eating fresh raw meat. He relates the story of the explorer Stefansson, who traveled the frozen Arctic with his col-

leagues living on fish, seal, polar bear, and caribou—
nothing else for nine months. Most of this was eaten raw,
and although undergoing the severest of hardships, they
were never sick.

On the return journey, they discovered a cache of
civilized food, including flour, preserved fruits and vegetables, and salted, cooked meat. Against Stefansson's
advice, the men ate this preserved food for several days.
They quickly developed diarrhea, loose teeth, and sore
mouths. Stefansson immediately placed them on raw
caribou tongue, and in a few days they were well.

But, who's going to eat raw beef, raw fish, or raw
chicken? Milk is by far the most convenient and acceptable
form of *raw animal protein* supplying the enzymes, antibodies, and nutrients needed for recovery from disease.

Dr. Crewe presented his findings on the therapeutic
uses of milk before the Minnesota State Medical Society
in 1923. His report was met with a veritable explosion of
apathy, indifference and, as Crewe had noted earlier, "almost to disrespect."

Dr. Crewe again reported on his work in 1930. He
quoted a colleague, who was also treating with raw milk,
"This was the worst case of psoriasis I have ever seen.
This boy was literally covered from head to foot with
scales. We put the boy on a milk diet and in less than a
month he had a skin like a baby's."

Crewe postulated, because of the remarkable effects
seen in such a great variety of diseases, that raw milk
may be supplying some hormonal elements to the patient. He repeatedly saw marked improvement in patients with toxic thyroid disease, a hormonal malady.

Dr. Crewe was especially enthusiastic about raw
milk in the treatment of disease of the prostate gland.
Rapid and marked improvement in the infection and in
the reduction of the size of the gland was seen routinely.
With shrinkage of the gland, the blockage will clear and
surgery can often be avoided, he reported. Urinary tract

infections, even without prostate swelling, are greatly improved by the treatment.

Many curious and unexpected results were obtained by Dr. Crewe "that could not be reasonably expected." Cardiac and kidney cases showed remarkable improvement. One patient with very advanced heart and kidney disease lost thirty pounds of fluid in six days.

On the treatment of high blood pressure, Crewe reported that he had "never seen such rapid and lasting results by any other method."

The milk treatment of diabetes was nothing short of phenomenal, most patients becoming sugar-free in four to ten weeks. This is astounding when you realize that five quarts of milk, the amount he used daily for diabetes, contains *one-half pound* of milk sugar.

Jim Redblood was our first diabetic to be treated with milk therapy. Jim was being treated at the Douglass Center for hardening of the arteries. His chelation therapy was working fine, but his diabetes suddenly went out of control. His blood sugar rose to well over 300 (three times normal). He had heard about my milk therapy and wanted to try it. He was willing to try anything within reason to avoid the inconvenience of daily insulin shots.*

He was put to bed and instructed to drink nothing but raw milk. That meant no water, absolutely nothing but the milk. His symptoms of diabetic acidosis—thirst, frequent urination, and vague abdominal pain—quickly abated. But, typical of patients on a milk fast, he complained of extreme weakness after about ten days. He was instructed to get a whole chicken, make a pot of chicken soup, and take a large bowl of it every evening, but continue on the milk fast otherwise. His strength rapidly returned.

---

* He was also well informed and aware that insulin shots may cause hardening of the arteries, the very condition we were treating.

On this program he lost weight which he needed to do, and his blood sugar returned to near normal levels. This is remarkable because milk contains large amounts of lactose, a form of sugar. We don't know why it works, but it does.*

And finally Crewe commented on that large group of patients for which no specific disease can be found. They used to be called "neuresthenics." In medical school they were half-joked about and called "crocks." They were diagnosed as having the "Triple 'P' Syndrome": Piss Poor Protoplasm.

Some of these unfortunate people are undoubtedly of weak and inferior constitution, and little can be done for them, especially if they are intellectually less than average. But the cruel appellation of "Triple 'P' Syndrome" should not be assumed until the nutritional factor has been thoroughly explored.

Crewe's classic description of these pathetic human beings is seen by every doctor, "These patients are often underweight. They may consume a fairly large amount of food, but they do not gain in weight or strength. They are often nervous and are frequently classed as neuresthenics. Usually, the skin condition is poor; they are sallow, and disappointed because no one can tell them what the trouble is. They do not respond well to medical treatment... Every physician knows this class of patients because they are unhappy and unsatisfactory to treat."

Crewe reported that they "respond admirably" to the milk therapy, but he added, "The chief fault of the treatment is that it is too simple... it does not appeal to the modern medical men."**

---

* We don't know why the chicken soup caused such a dramatic increase in energy either, but can 10,000,000 Jewish mothers be wrong?

** This was 1929. You can imagine how they would snicker today.

J.E. Crewe, M.D., a determined and dedicated physician, left no doubt of his stand on milk therapy, "...the treatment of various diseases over a period of eighteen years with a practically exclusive milk diet has convinced me personally that *the most important single factor in the cause of disease and in the resistance to disease is food.* I have seen so many instances of the rapid and marked response to this form of treatment that nothing could make me believe this is not so..."

While the fat fighters have been pushing skim milk and peanut oil, Dr. Alan Howard, Cambridge University, England, has discovered that whole milk actually *protects* against abnormally high cholesterol. Feeding two quarts of whole milk a day to volunteers caused a drop in cholesterol. Butter caused an increase in cholesterol.*

Dr. George Mann, Vanderbilt University School of Medicine, concurs with Dr. Howard. He found that four quarts of whole milk per day will lower the blood cholesterol level by twenty-five percent. Cambridge's Howard concluded, "...all this business that saturated fats in milk are bad for you is a lot of nonsense."**

Human milk also has tremendous potential as a curative agent. Breast milk is the only known mammalian source of lenolenic acid. Lenolenic acid is essential for prostaglandin synthesis, and prostaglandins do wonderful things for you. They prevent arthritis, (or halt the course of existing arthritis). They keep your blood from clotting. They normalize weight, work against cancer, and alleviate premenstrual syndrome.

---

* That doesn't mean that butter is bad for you. There is *absolutely no proof* that a temporary rise in cholesterol is harmful.

** Sure beats taking clofibrate, a chemical prescribed by doctors for lowering the cholesterol level of the blood. Clofibrate can cause heart attacks, gall bladder attacks and cancer.

People used to think John D. Rockerfeller was crazy for drinking fresh human milk on a regular basis. He was way ahead of his time and lived to the age of 86.*

Because of advances in immunology, milk therapy took a great step forward in the second half of the 20th century. It has been known since the earliest days of husbandry that the newborn calf cannot survive without the milk produced by its mother. This initial milk, called colostrum, was a mystery until the science of immunology revealed the secrets of the udder, or mammary gland.

Colostrum is the milk secreted by an animal (or human) before and just after delivery of the young. This special milk, which greatly resembles blood under the microscope, continues to be produced for about a week after delivery of the calf. *It is the most nutrient-packed food known to man.* Yet until recently, it was considered unfit for human consumption!

One early twentieth century textbook on food products,[3] written by qualified scientists, listed colostrum under "abnormal milk." They said of colostrum, "The secretion from the udders of cows and other mammals, for some days after the birth of the young, acts as a purgative and has a pungent taste. It is called 'colostrum,' and is not considered fit for human food."

The authors of this text obviously had never tasted colostrum but were merely repeating the folklore of that period. Colostrum has no "purgative" action, and it does not have a "pungent taste." It tastes like what it is—very rich milk.

Colostrum has ten to seventeen times the iron content of regular milk. It contains ten times more Vitamin A and three times as much Vitamin D. Many of the important minerals are more concentrated in colostrum. I used to take a handful of vitamins and minerals every day. I now drink a half-pint of colostrum twice daily and take no additional vitamins and minerals.

---

*He died rich.

But the most important ingredient of colostrum is its antibodies. The newborn calf is highly susceptible to life-threatening infections. The colostrum milk has a high concentration of antibodies that protect the baby calf. Without this colostrum with its protective antibodies, the newborn calf simply won't make it.

It is very easy to prove that the immune substances, called antibodies, found in early mother's milk are a "survival package" for the young calf. If two calves are born at the same time, and one is fed directly from the mother, the other from a lactating cow that has not recently delivered, the calf not given his mother's milk will die within two months. The calf getting his mother's antibody-packed colostrum milk will survive even if born in a sleet storm!

Scientists interested in treating disease without powerful chemicals postulated that if this potent colostrum milk can shield the young calf against practically all bacterial, viral, and fungal disease, perhaps it could be used to treat diseases in humans. The "experts" of the day, including the American Medical Association and prominent professors, said that this was "contrary to recognized theories" on treatment, and besides, it had been "proven" that antibodies could not be absorbed from the stomach and intestine after the first few days of life.

Scientific history is replete with examples of investigators not realizing that what they had discovered was discovered years ago. This was understandable before computer science transformed the library into a veritable model of efficiency in information gathering. Burrows and Haven, in 1948, were amazed to find that milk transferred immunity, which Ehrlich and Klemperer had proven in 1892.[4] In spite of their work, clumsy and confusing research at the time discredited Burrows and Haven, setting immune milk research back thirty years.

The discovery and rediscovery that antibodies can be absorbed when taken by mouth was of colossal importance. It opened the way for a simpler and safer mode of treatment of diseases—the milk therapy of Hippocrates and Crewe made a hundred times more effective by hyperimmunization of milk.

Carrying on this eighty-year fight for immune milk therapy, Doctors Peterson and Campbell of the University of Minnesota began rekindling the fires of controversy in 1955. Writing in the prestigious British journal, Lancet, they showed conclusively, through a scholarly review of the literature and their own brilliant research that:

1) Antibody against disease is absorbed from the gastrointestinal tract into the blood.

2) Rheumatoid arthritis and hay fever will respond to immune milk therapy.

3) The udder acts as an antibody-forming organ independent of the cow's blood-immune system. The appropriate bacteria, fungus, or virus need only be infused directly into the teat canal for antibody production in the colostrum milk.

Peterson remarked in a speech before the Chicago Farmer's Club that their findings on the absorption of antibody from milk were "largely on the basis of a hunch."[5] The medical literature for the past twenty years had stated emphatically that the wall of the gastrointestinal tract was not permeable to immune globulin (antibodies). All the work by great men of science such as Paul Ehrlich, done in the late 1 9th and early 20th centuries, had been neglected by "modern science." Fortunately for millions of suffering people, Peterson and Campbell looked back into history, learned from it, and followed their "hunch."

The reactionary American Medical Association, in spite of eighty years of confirmatory research from Ehrlich to Peterson on the efficacy of immune milk therapy, has either forgotten or ignored this therapy at different periods in time. The Arthritis and Rheumatism Foundation, always antagonistic toward anything but

conventional chemical approaches to arthritis, announced that "accepted medical theory" disagreed with
the Peterson findings. A representative of the National
Office of the Arthritis and Rheumatism Foundation reported that some doctors in Tucson, Arizona "had made
a study" using immune milk and found it had no effect
on rheumatism or arthritis.[6]

Things got so emotional in Virginia that this perfectly harmless food was impounded by the state from
two dairies.[7] They said it was a "biological product" (no
kidding) and needed a Federal license. The Food and
Drug Administration, having the typical bureaucratic
mind and an instinct for control rather than common
sense, declared that immune milk is a drug and confis-
cated eighty cases.[8]

Although less extensive than his work on arthritis,
Peterson's work with allergies is no less impressive. The
cow's udder was stimulated with pollen antigen such as rag
weed. The resulting immune milk was fed to asthma and
hay fever sufferers. In a controlled experiment, thirty-six patients were improved to a significant degree. The symptoms
disappeared in a definite order: First, the asthma, then nasal
congestion, and last, itching of the eyes.

Perhaps the disease least likely to be cured by immune milk (or anything else) is multiple sclerosis. Dr.
Donald H. Hastings, a Bismarck, North Dakota veterinarian, is a product of the University of Minnesota and so
was aware of the pioneer work of Peterson and Campbell
on immune milk.

Hastings read that the Japanese had isolated measles
virus from the intestines of multiple sclerosis patients.
Knowing that Peterson had had success treating rheumatoid arthritis patients with immune milk from cows immunized with streptococcus antigen, he postulated that
multiple sclerosis is a viral-induced disease caused by
measles and other viruses. He produced immune milk
from measles-innoculated cows and fed the milk to mul-

tiple sclerosis victims. Hastings reported that forty percent of the multiple sclerosis patients got relief including
alleviation of numbness, decrease in muscle twitching,
and less fatigue.

As would be expected, the Multiple Sclerosis Society
was not enthusiastic about Hastings' report and deemed
it "placebo effect." But Hastings countered with the observation that hyperimmune colostrum milk and regular
colostrum taste and look the same, but, "We put people
on plain colostrum, and it doesn't work. I don't know
what's going on, but I know hyperimmune milk works. .
. If I had multiple sclerosis I'd take it."[9]

Milk has been used for gastric disorders, especially ulcers, for centuries. In the 19th century, Cruvelheir advocated
milk as the most important part of the treatment of gastric
ulcer.[10] Later, Sippy popularized the continuous use of milk,
and the Sippy Diet has been the standard treatment for gastric and duodenal ulcers for generations.

Milk also contains an anti-viral agent. British studies[11] have shown that some mysterious substance in the
aqueous portion of the milk, below the cream layer,
works against virus infections.* Formula and boiled milk
do not contain this virus-fighting agent.

But with the tinkering of milk, homogenization and
pasteurization, this highly effective, simple and safe
treatment for many of our most common ailments has become a dangerous two-edged sword. We now know that
while curing the ulcers, we have been giving the patients
heart attacks! (See Chapter III)

Benjamin M. Bernstein, M.D., a gastroenterologist,
described a much more difficult gastrointestinal disease,
"...very sick with active diarrhea, abdominal pain, loss of
blood and consequent anemia, frequently with fever,
markedly dehydrated and in severe cases, 'nigh unto

---

*It is in a heat-stable macromolecule, but we don't know what it is.

death'."[12] Bernstein enthusiastically recommended raw milk in the treatment of this disease, ulcerative colitis.

It would appear to this writer that colitis would be helped by treating with milk at the other end. Milk soothes the lining of the stomach and duodenum. Why would it not do the same for the lining of an inflamed colon? We have searched the literature, and find no reference to this mode of therapy for colitis. We will pursue it.

Bernstein was so enthusiastic about the use of raw milk for the treatment of gastrointestinal disease that he said, "...milk not only may, but should be used in the management of *any type or variety* of gastrointestinal disorder. "[13]

There is hardly a specialty in medicine that has not in the past successfully used raw milk for therapy. Samuel Zuerling, M.D., ear, nose, and throat specialist, Assistant Surgeon, Brooklyn Eye and Ear Hospital, reported an unusual case treated with raw milk.[14] "Not long ago a gentleman came to me for relief of a severe burning sensation in the nose, stating, 'Doctor, my nose feels like it is on fire.' This poor gentleman was more than extremely uncomfortable—he was panicky. He had sought relief and obtained no results... the patient readily acceded to a milk... diet and in a few days had complete and permanent relief."

Relief of muscle cramps in pregnancy was reported by John Fowler, M.D., Worcester, Massachusetts. He said the raw milk therapy was "very effective, and in no instance where used faithfully, were the muscle cramps in pregnant women a cause of discomfort."

James A. Tobey, Doctor of Public Health, Chief of Health Services for the Borden Company, wrote about the use of raw milk in the treatment and prevention of worms in humans.[15] Dr. Tobey's description of these intestinal and blood invaders is frightening: "The worms that plague us include such dangerous invaders as the hookworm, the trichina, the filaria, and the flukes, and such uncomfortable and troublesome guests as the tapeworm, the round worm, the thread worm, and many others. Once implanted in the intestines, some of these guests not only are very difficult to evict, but they may give rise to symptoms that resemble those of typhoid fever, cholera, and even appendicitis, and they may cause diarrhea and colic and sometimes anemia."

Although sanitation is the first line of defense against these repulsive little visitors, that is, don't get them in the first place, milk is another effective defense. We know that they flourish on starch but have a tough time surviving on protein. And casein, the principle protein of milk, is particularly destructive to the parasite. Hegner proved experimentally that a diet consisting largely of the protein casein will often lead to a total elimination of the worms. To milk's other therapeutic virtues we can add that of vermifuge—a killer of worms.[16]

P.I.D. would be about the last thing in the world you would expect to be cured by milk. P.I.D. stands for Pelvic Inflammatory Disease in women. But that doesn't really tell you what it is. P.I.D. means "pus tubes." It's an abscess of pus involving the fallopian tube and ovary—a nasty mess. It used to be a disease of the downtrodden, usually caused by gonorrhea. But P.I.D. has moved up in the social scale, thanks to the I.U.D. contraceptive device.

Seaman reported a case of P.I.D. treated in India with raw milk.[17] Conventional antibiotic therapy had not helped. She went to an Indian country doctor who treated her with raw milk *straight from his cow* and herbs cooked in raw milk. In six weeks she was free of disease.

I know I would be laughed out of town if I tried it, but I would like to hook up a lukemia patient directly to the teat of a cow producing colostrum. It would also be interesting to see what it would do for an A.I.D.S. victim.

At the Douglass Center in Atlanta we have rediscovered the wheel for the fourth time. Hippocrates, Ehrlich, and Peterson were absolutely right. Raw milk, especially hyperimmune raw colostrum milk, is a great therapeutic agent against many diseases.

Destin Callahan got off to a bad start in life. He was not breast fed. Asthma developed by the time he was six months old. His mother couldn't recall any time during his nine years that he hasn't wheezed. He has been in and out of hospitals with asthma attacks, sometimes nearly fatal, at least six times every year. He has been dosed with antibiotics and cortisone almost continuously since the age of six months. Destin is nine years old, but he is the physical size of a six year old. He is bright but thin and delicate.

Destin's mother and father came to the Douglass Center desperate to try something different and non-toxic. They felt, and justifiably so, that Destin's poor growth was at least partially due to constant medication.

He had been to many allergists with frequent skin testing. We decided to have a serum manufactured containing the various factors to which Destin was allergic by skin test. This serum was then injected into a pregnant cow. After the calf was born, the colostrum was taken from the mother, frozen, and given daily to Destin.* His parents had been told that their son was allergic to milk. He was allergic only to pasteurized milk.

After six weeks of therapy, Destin began to improve, and for the first time in his life he stopped wheezing. His parents were astounded and almost afraid to believe what they were seeing. But, Christmas Eve their hopes were dashed. Destin, excited about Christmas, had a severe asthmatic attack.

Marcy and Les Callahan were by now convinced that immune colostrum therapy was the answer for their son. Having the courage as well as the conviction, they eschewed the customary medications and gave Destin colostrum every hour. The massive antibody attack of the colostrum turned the tide, and by Christmas morning, Destin was completely without

---

* The calf was named "Destin" and a picture of the calf, with his name on a plaque around his neck, was given to him.

symptoms. What a Christmas present for this young man who had hardly ever known a well day!

The Effect of Milk on Growth

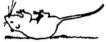
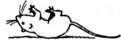
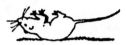

No milk, Died at age of 7 weeks | One-fifth teaspoon of milk a day. Died at age of 7 weeks, 1 day. | Two-fifths teaspoon of milk a day. Died at age of 7 weeks, 3 days.

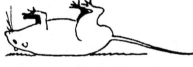
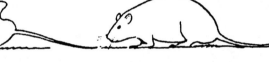

Three-fifths teaspoon of milk a day. Weight, 150 grams at 24 weeks old. Died at 32 weeks of age.

One teaspoon of milk a day. Weight, 175 grams at 24 weeks old.

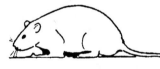
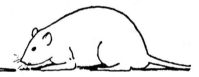

One and one-fifth teaspoon of milk a day. Weight, 190 grams at 24 weeks old.

One and three-fifths teaspoon of milk a day. Weight, 210 grams at 24 weeks old.

Milk probably contains growth factors that haven't been discovered. Destin grew rapidly after starting the raw milk and colostrum treatment. An experiment done with rats way back in 1927 vividly illustrated the remarkable growing power of even a small amount of milk.

The rats were given a very good diet except the milk portion was very carefully controlled. They could eat all they wanted except for the milk. The above illustration is from a March, 1928 publication reporting the phenomenal findings of the experiment.

Although human milk and human colostrum are without a doubt the perfect food for healthy babies, cow's colostrum may actually be better than human milk during illness. A protein fraction in the blood called IGG is the main protective agent of the blood system. Human colostrum contains 2% IGG for disease protection. But cow's colostrum contains a phenomenal amount of IGG: 86%.[18]

It's a sad commentary on modern medicine that this powerful and safe therapeutic agent, which can be produced at moderate cost, cannot be obtained readily except in the state of Nevada and Atlanta, Georgia. The rest of it, except for that gotten by the suckling calf, is simply thrown away.

But milk is not for everyone. Africans literally starving to death have been known to throw away gifts of American powdered milk because it harbored evil spirits.* Colombian indians, on the other hand, kept asking for more.** It gave the Navajo indians diarrhea so they threw it out.***

The worst case of misguided milkfare took place in Northeast Brazil. Milk was given to the starving natives. They were extremely deficient in Vitamin A. The rapid growth caused by the milk led to an even more extreme vitamin A deficiency which caused irreversible blindness.[19] It was just too much of a good thing.

Yet, not all dark-skinned people are intolerant to milk. The Bahimas of Africa drink six pints a day. In fact, they eat little else.****

---

* They were absolutely correct.

** They were using it to whitewash their huts.

*** They didn't have any huts to paint.

**** This is also true of the Nuers of the Upper Nile, the Todas, the Kazaks, and the Hottentots. There are others, but you never heard of them.

We'll end this chapter with an interesting quote from an unexpected source:

"Milk sounds like patent medicines when all its virtues are catalogued. It is the oldest prescription for the building of strong, healthy bodies; Nature's revitalizer; Nature's maker of rich, red blood; Nature's nerve quieter, Nature's antidote for that tired feeling.

"If milk were put up in bottles of different shapes and sizes, if it were given fanciful names and announced for what it really is— the greatest body builder and health restorer in the world— people would flock to buy it at fancy prices; but because it costs so little and is delivered every morning at our doorstep we seldom give its virtues a thought."

Metropolitan Life Insurance Company, 1921[20]

REFERENCES

1. Certified Milk Magazine, January 1929.

2. Ibid.

3. Food Products—*Their Source, Chemistry and Use,* pp. 387, Bailey & Bailey, Glakiston, Philadelphia, 1928.

4. Journal of Immune Milk, Volume I, Nr.1, June 1964, *Immune Milk*, pp. 3 -28.

5. Transcript of Speech delivered before Chicago Farmer's Club, April 6, 1959.

6. The Milk Dealer, June 1960.

7. Ibid.

8. Dairy Records, November 1980.

9. DVM, February 1981.

10. B.M. Bernstein, Paper presented to the AAMMC Conference, Atlantic City, New Jersey, June 8,1942.

11. Matthews, et al, The Lancet, December 25,1976, pp. 1387.

12. Loc. cit.

13. Loc. cit.

14. Certified Milk Magazine, September 1936.

15. Ibid., April, 1935.

16. Science, 75:225, February 20, 1932; JAMA, April 9, 1932; JAMA 83:83, 1924.

17. Seaman, *Women and the Crisis in Sex Hormones,* Bantam Books, 1979, pp. 203.

18. Bunce, C.E., Natural History, February 1969.

19. Certified Milk Magazine, November/December, 1946.

20. Metropolitan Life Insurance Company, 1921.

Chapter XII

LET 'EM EAT STEAK*

"I like meat and have little faith in dieticians."
Earnest A. Hooton, Ph.D., Jc.D.
Professor of Anthropology, Harvard

Vegetarianism vs. Omnivorism

If you are one of the six million American vegetarians reading this book, you're not going to like this part. If you are sensitive, skip to page 230.

The anti-red meat vegetarians say that most meat is contaminated. They're probably right, but so are vegetables. Yes, the vegetarians say, but one can wash the contaminants off vegetables and fruits, and you can't with red meat.

What they seem to forget is that a great deal of the insecticides sprayed on plants goes into the soil and is then taken up within the tissues of the plant. You can't wash that away either.** At least the animal has a liver to detoxify poisons. Plants do not. So why pick on red meat?

At the Douglass Center we assume that everything*** is contaminated, and so we put all of our patients on a purified garlic preparation that neutralizes many contaminants. For even further protection, we use a lot of Vitamin E and Vitamin C.

Periodically America goes through an anti-meat, anti-fat crusade. In 1926 a small but vociferous group

---

   * With apologies to Marie Antoinette.

   ** Did you know that in 1977 the FDA found that *half the southeastern corn crop* was contaminated with aflatoxin? It is also found in pasteurized milk and peanut butter. Aflatoxin is highly carcinogenic.

  *** Except raw certified milk.

proclaimed that meat and fat caused kidney disease, arthritis, and high blood pressure.[1] Part of this was undoubtedly the continuing Puritanical concept in our country that anything as good tasting as meat and fat must be bad for you. But the explorer Stefansson's experiments with meat and fat in the Arctic, which we will describe subsequently, wrote a new chapter in nutrition. A lot of brilliant theories against meat faded into nothingness. Sixty years later the anti-meat doomsayers are at it again.

I'm tired of vegetarians telling me that the bible says don't eat meat. There are at least a dozen references in the bible advocating the eating of meat and the fat of meat. They're in Appendix VI. I'll quote one extremely interesting passage from *Timothy* I because you probably won't look at the appendix:

"Now the Spirit speaketh expressly that in the latter times some shall depart from the faith, giving heed to seducing spirits, and doctrines of devils . . . Forbidding to marry, and commanding to abstain from meats which God hath created to be received with thanksgiving of them which believe and know the truth."

According to the anthropologists, man was a meat-eater long before he took up Caesar salad. And if you think man ascended from the ape, then there is further proof that humans have always been carniverous. It has always been assumed that primates were strictly vegetarians. Nothing could be further from the truth. Goodall[2] studied apes in their natural habitat and discovered that they eat meat on a regular basis. Baboons eat vervet monkeys and other small animals. Chimpanzees eat small baboons. They love it.

The National Zoo in Washington attempted to breed Amazonian monkeys. They were fed a total fruit diet and nothing happened.* Within weeks of feeding meat to the monkeys, normal mating took place and many healthy babies were born.

An interesting aside about lions: although they are definite carnivores, they are choosy. They seldom attack and eat humans, even little ones.** Leakey[3] observed lions walking through his camp at night sniffing at humans asleep. They could have easily attacked and eaten them. But they would sniff and walk away, apparently not liking the smell of humans.***

Archeological studies have shown that Cro-Magnon man ate bear, lion, hyenas, wild horse, and the wooly rhinocerous.**** In America the paleolithic Homo sapiens ate the wolf, beaver, and the American camel.*****

In China, Peking Man was found to have lunched on camel, deer, elephant and ostrich.****** Neanderthals not only ate the wooly rhinocerous, but the 12 -foot auroch.*******

There is no society in the world that is entirely vegetarian. The Hindus of India come closest. Dr. H. Leon Abrams[4] reports on India, "...the greater percentage of the population, who subsist almost entirely on vegetable foods, suffer from kwashiokor, other forms of malnutrition, and have the shortest life span in the world."********

---

* Actually, a *lot* happened, (you know monkeys) but there were no pregnancies.

** Alligators will eat little humans (or anything else).

*** You probably don't either.

**** The *wooly rhinocerous*?

***** You don't see many of those any more.

****** It tastes terrible.

******* The 12-foot auroch couldn't fly, and the Neanderthals ate them right out of existence.[5]

******** They'll probably never win the Superbowl.

There are a lot of vegetarian countries, but none of them seem to accomplish much.*

The Aztecs were carnivorous too. They ate *each other.* By the beginning of the 1 6th century they were butchering 250 thousand men a year![6] They would rip out his heart** then butcher and eat the rest.***

During the entire paleolithic period, man spent most of his time looking for meat. According to Johnson,[7] humans have been on earth "for at least three to four million years." Abrams says[8] that "For all but the last 10,000 years, or over 99% of this time span..." man was exclusively a meat eater except for the gathering of fruits and nuts when available.

So don't believe that stuff about primitive man being a veggie. The Australopithecenes would laugh in your face.****

Is today's human so different that he can thrive on fruits and vegetables where Cro-Magnon Man and the ancient Egyptians***** couldn't? Maybe we should take a closer look at the modern vegetarian. If you're tired of this and convinced that you should drink raw milk or eat some other form of animal protein, skip over to page 230.

The diets of 119 strict vegetarians in eighty households in Israel were studied at the Hebrew University. All of these vegetarians were deficient in the essential amino acids methionine and tryptophan.[10]

Babies fed a strict vegetarian diet, meaning, of course, no milk but just fruits and vegetables, do not grow at a normal rate. They get short-changed on B12, folic acid, zinc, calories, proteins, calcium and riboflavin (B2).[11] Even a

---

* Show me a vegetarian country, and I'll show you a loser.

** There were no anesthesiologists.

*** This was, ostensibly, sacrifice to the gods. No one messed with a priest. He always got the best cuts.

**** So would homo erectus (including those in San Francisco).

***** The Egyptians used to dilute their milk with urine. It made it go farther.[9]

breast-fed baby may become malnourished if the mother has been a true vegetarian for a number of years.[12]

The Seventh Day Adventists are often cited as a good example of why you shouldn't eat meat. They have much less heart disease and cancer. But they eat plenty of dairy products and eggs, and they don't use tobacco, alcohol, coffee, tea, or cola beverages.*

Puerto Ricans, unlike the Seventh Day Adventists, eat large amounts of pork.** Yet, they have a very low rate of colon cancer and breast cancer.***[13]

In case you read that last ***, don't get me wrong. I have nothing against Seventh Day Adventists.****

Eggs have been catching it too because of their high cholesterol content. We have said a lot about cholesterol, but we can't stop without mentioning the findings of famous heart surgeon Michael DeBakey. He analyzed 1700 patients with hardening of the arteries and found that there was no correlation between blood cholesterol levels and the degree of atherosclerosis.[14]

The prestigious New England Journal of Medicine[15] had a report on eggs and cholesterol. A group of New Guinea natives, whose diet is exceedingly low in cholesterol, were fed eggs to measure the cholesterol-raising effect of eggs. They figured the serum cholesterol levels would be blown off the charts. The eggs had no significant effect on the blood cholesterol.

Another study done by the American Cancer Society[16] revealed that non-egg users had a higher death rate from heart attacks and strokes than egg users. This was a very large (and so convincing) study involving over 800,000 people.

---

* What do they do for fun?

** Pork would be the perfect meat if it wasn't for trichinosis. Why can't they produce a trichinosis-free pork?

*** They also have a lot of fun.

**** My son, William Campbell Douglass, III, is an SDA. He's a good kid, a definite improvement over his father.

After a heart attack, the cardiologist will inevitably place the patient on a low-cholesterol, low-fat diet, thus making him even more miserable. This type of diet is delicious to grazing animals but not to omnivorous humans.

The Medical Research Council of Great Britain in 1968 did a study in which the fate of patients put on a low saturated fat diet after a heart attack was determined and compared to patients on a high saturated fat diet. They concluded that the unsaturated fat diet had no effect on the ultimate course of the patients. The number of second heart attacks and deaths were the same in both groups. Two other studies, one done in Oslo, Norway and one in England, came to the same conclusion.

Professor H. Leon Abrams, Jr. sums it up,[17] "Any one who deliberately avoids cholesterol in his diet may be inadvertenty courting heart disease."*

Abrams also pointed out that meat, being a much more concentrated protein than plant protein requires two-thirds less time to eat and requires much less time to prepare. He said, "By eating as much meat as they could secure, the Austrolopithecenes... had more free time."**[18]

A few more hits on the vegetarians, and we'll move on.

Tooth decay isn't caused entirely by drinking pasteurized milk and eating sugar. A strictly vegetarian diet will do it too. Throughout the paleolithic period when humans subsisted primarily on meat, tooth decay was a rarity. As humans went agricultural, tooth decay increased.[19]

Eskimos and Icelanders are more recent examples. The Eskimos, who are aboriginal, and the Icelanders, who are European, remained free of cavities until they abandoned their fish and meat diet.[20]

---

* What Professor Abrams is saying in a nice way is that the American Heart Association is giving lousy advice on nutrition.
** For other pursuits, such as playing cards and frollicking around.

The Director of the National Museum in Iceland says that it is definitely established that during 600 years, 1200 to 1800 in Iceland, there were *no dental cavities.* The foods they ate were milk and milk products, mutton, beef and fish. The ate *no carbohydrate.* The only exception to this was a little moss soup in the summer, but this was a rare "fun food" of little nutritional importance.

Two Indian tribes reveal the same thing. The prehistoric Indians of California were vegetarians, unlike most folks of that period, and they had tooth decay. In contrast, the Sioux Indians lived on buffalo meat and were devoid of cavities.[21] The Pueblos worshipped the Corn God, but he was not grateful. They have the most wretched teeth of all of the American Indian tribes. They live on corn, squash and beans. The Laplanders, who ate mostly reindeer meat during the 18th century, rarely had cavities. Modern Laps have a decay rate of 85%[22] of their teeth.

The most overrated profession today, except doctors in general, is probably dental hygiene, and the biggest waste of money is toothpaste, dental floss, tooth brushes, and waterpicks. Stefansson puts the case very colorfully, "Teeth superior on the average to those of the presidents of our largest toothpaste companies are found in the world today, and have existed during past ages, among people who violate every precept of current dentifrice advertising...The best teeth and the healthiest mouths were found among people who never drank milk since they ceased to be suckling babes and who never in their lives tasted or tested any of the other things which we usually recommend for sound teeth... They never took any pains to cleanse their teeth or mouths. They did not visit their dentist twice a year or even once in a lifetime... so far as an extensive correspondence with authorities has yet been able to show, a complete absence of tooth decay from entire populations has never existed in the past, and does not exist now, except where meat is either exclusive or heavily predominant in the diet."[23]

If you feel weak on a pure vegetarian diet, I'll tell you why. Venison (deer meat) contains 572 *calories* per 100 grams of weight. One hundred grams of fruit or vegetable only contains a lousy *100 calories*. In other words, you have to eat almost *six times* more by weight if you are strictly vegetarian.*

Some vegetarians condemn meat because it contains cadaverine.** But we now know that this misnamed substance is not only harmless, but essential to normal function of the brain and the rest of the nervous system.[24]

Remember that we're not criticizing all vegetarians, but only the purists who eat *no form* of animal protein, (milk, eggs, cheese, beef, fish, etc.). You don't have to eat "red meat." It's just silly not to.*** If you have religious prohibitions against meat, then you must eat eggs, cheese, and milk.

The overemphasis of unsaturated fats in the American diet, and vegetarians particularly, may lead to a brand new disease epidemic in the next 10 - 20 years. It is called Ceroid Storage Disease.[25]

Ceroid is a wax-like pigment that is formed from the heating of unsaturated fatty acids. It's called polymerization and you may ploymerize yourself to an early grave if you get too fanatic about vegetarianism.

Let's look at a typical case of this new disease. A young man came to the emergency room complaining of bellyache. The operation revealed a spleen filled with ceroid. His history was interesting. He had been fed soy bean milk as an infant. As an adult he followed a strict vegetarian diet for religious reasons. This diet consisted of soy bean and wheat protein cooked in corn and Wesson oil. A perfect setup for ceroid storage disease. As

---

    * You'll never make it.

    ** Yipes, sounds like gas from a corpse.

    *** Most vegetarians I know will eat a steak if someone else is picking up the check.

pure vegetarianism becomes more popular, ceroid storage disease may become more common.*

Research at the University of Georgia on various fats helped to exonerate "red meat."[26] They found that adding stearate fat (from animals) to the diet of rats lowered cholesterol levels. Vegetable fats had no effect. The stearate also lowered blood pressure.**

The observations of the great explorer, Vilhjalmur Stefansson,[27] on raw meat and raw fish as a complete diet are pertinent to our subject.*** His findings are totally opposite to modern nutritional thinking. Here's what Stefansson said, "In 1906 I went to the arctic with the food tastes and beliefs of the average American. By 1918, after eleven years as an Eskimo among Eskimos, I had learned things which caused me to shed most of those beliefs."

Stefansson catalogued the dietary "truths" of 1935, which are still believed to be true today by practically all schools of nutrition:

- To be healthy you need a varied diet composed of elements from both the animal and vegetable kingdoms.
- Eating the same thing daily for prolonged periods causes a revulsion against that food.
- One must eat fruit for a "balanced" diet.
- One must eat vegetables for a "balanced" diet.

---

* Then again, it may not. Only time will tell.

** But these studies will have to be repeated. They were financed by the National Dairy Council and the National Livestock and Meat Board.

*** I *know* raw meat and raw fish are not raw milk, but all three are *raw animal protein* and where Stefansson says "raw meat" or "raw fish", you can substitute "raw milk". This is *vital* to your understanding of the importance of raw milk in your diet.

- Nuts and coarse grains are necessary.

- Certain harmful bacteria will flourish in the intestine if you eat too much meat.

- The less meat you eat the better. It will cause arthritis, hardening of the arteries, high blood pressure, and a calcium deficiency.

- You should, in fact, be a vegetarian.

- Without fruits or vegetables, especially fruits, you will get scurvy.

- Man cannot live on meat alone. Your kidneys will stop working.

Stefansson proved that all of these views are incorrect. He ridiculed them, especially the prohibition on eating meat, "There would be protein poisoning and, in general, hell to pay," he said, with tongue in cheek.

Living with various Eskimo tribes, Stefansson ate raw fish for breakfast, raw fish for lunch, and boiled fish for dinner. He became quite fond of this one food diet and even learned to eat the greatest of Eskimo delicacies - raw, rotten fish! "About the fourth month of my first Eskimo winter," he remarked, "I was looking forward to every meal (rotten or fresh) . . . Civilized people eat decayed milk products (sour cream) and decayed cheese," he said, "so why not decayed fish?"*

I tried rotten shark in Iceland. Once you get it past your nose, it tastes pretty good. On the north coast of Iceland, they still eat rotten eggs. In the old days, they ate rotten sheep heads.[28]

---

* Never eat rotten fish in the summer. The Eskimos say it's bad for you. Eat it frozen—tastes like a ripe cheese.

Stefansson, living on fish and water for a year, did not get scurvy. In all, he lived in the Arctic for five years exclusively on fish and meat, mostly raw, and remained in perfect health.

Whenever the men of the expedition were exposed to civilized cooking, they would get indigestion, headache and feel miserable. In most cases, they would be happy to get back on the meat diet.

Critics of Stefansson said that maybe it was okay in the frigid temperatures of the artic under extreme physical conditions, but one would certainly die eating nothing but meat under modern sedentary conditions. But the Institute of American Meat Packers believed in Stefansson* and donated the funds, no strings attached, to authenticate or refute the explorer's amazing and completely unorthodox views on nutrition.

Six prestigious institutions were represented on the scientific committee: The American Museum of Natural History, Cornell University Medical College, Harvard University, Johns Hopkins University, Russell Sage Institute of Pathology, and the University of Chicago. A meat packer's representative and Stefansson were also on the committee. The study was directed by the dietetic ward of Bellevue Hospital, New York City.

Many vegetarians eat eggs and drink milk and still consider themselves vegetarians. Although this is illogical, Stefansson said he would also be illogical and exclude them—nothing but meat, period.

One leading European authority assured the researchers very solemnly that the experiment would not last a week. He had tried the experiment himself, he said, and it was quite preposterous to think that a man could live on nothing but meat for a week, much less an entire year. Other scientists said that the two subjects, Stefansson

---

*Naturally.

and Karsten Anderson, another explorer, would die within fifteen days of the onset of the experiment.

Stefansson and Anderson thrived on the diet, winter and summer. Their stamina increased with the lengthening of the meat period. Stefansson remarked that he had never felt more energetic or optimistic. It is common knowledge that the Eskimos are the happiest people in the world when in their primitive state. Stefansson maintains that this may be due to their exclusively meat diet.*

Inexplicably, Stefansson became ill on the second day of the experiment. It was inexplicable to everyone but Stefansson. The critics were smirking. Stefansson had warned them that meat without fat was an incomplete food.** After a few days of fat sirloin and brains fried in bacon fat, he was entirely well. Stefansson warned, "If yours is a meat diet, then you simply must have fat with your lean; otherwise you would sicken and die."

Arctic tribes are connoisseurs of fats the way civilized westerners are connoisseurs of wines. The marrow of the long bones is considered the finest of delicacies.*** Also held in high esteem is the fat around the kidneys and behind the eyeball.

Contrary to what you have heard, (and what I was taught in medical school), you can eat polar bear liver. About one time in six, according to Stefansson, it will give you a headache but there is no record of man or beast dying from eating polar bear liver.

I use meat as a reducing diet in my practice. I had one patient, 5 feet tall, who weighed well over two hundred pounds to whom I suggested the all-meat diet. I

---

* Reminder: Raw milk, in place of raw meat, will have the same effect.

** Just as skim milk is an incomplete food with the milk fat taken away.

*** Except moose nose—that's the greatest. They eat it boiled.

didn't think that she believed me and would try the diet. When she returned to my office three months later, I didn't recognize her. She had lost well over fifty pounds and thought I was a magician.*

I found out years later that the DuPont company had used a similar program on their executives with great success. Their diet was 70% fat and meat with the other 30% for a small amount of baked potato, fresh fruit or salad. It was reported at the time, "The reducing of the corpulent proved painless, even pleasant, some said they were going to stick to the diet permanently."[29]

Stefansson was overweight at the beginning of the all-meat diet but quickly lost it. Eskimos, he pointed out, are never fat when left on their native diet of meat, "When you see Eskimos in their native garments you do get the impression of fat round faces, or fat round bodies; but the roundness of face is a racial peculiarity and the rest of the effect is produced by loose and puffy garments. See them stripped and you do not find the abdominal protuberances and folds which are so numerous at Coney Island beaches and so persuasive in arguments against nudism."

Raw milk and kefir, in spite of their sugar and fat content, can also be used effectively for weight reduction. This method is more acceptable than the meat diet to most people and so it is generally more successful.**

Although raw milk doesn't contain enough Vitamin C, according to the U.S. Government and nutrition experts, to supply the daily minimum needed, people on a undiluted raw milk diet don't get scurvy.*** This is probably because of greater "bioavailability"**** of the Vita-

---

* I was more astounded than she was, but I didn't let her know it.
** Cheaper, too.
*** Babies are different. See Chapter IX.
**** The ability of the body to absorb the particular nutrient in question from the digestive tract.

min C in raw milk. Or the natural Vitamin C may be more potent, thus requiring less of it for good health.

Stefansson's study of Iceland confirms that milk and meat can keep you free of scurvy (Vitamin C deficiency) and other diseases just as well as fruits and vegetables can.[30] When the Irish discovered Iceland in 700 A.D.,* they were forced onto a very strict diet of milk, milk products, and fish. Stefansson arrived 1200 years later, in 1905, to study the Icelanders, past and present. He collected the bones and skulls from an abandoned medieval graveyard and took them to Harvard. These ancient people, who rarely if ever ate fruits and vegetables, showed no sign of scurvy.

Doctors decided in the 18th century that fruits, especially limes, prevented and cured scurvy. Dr. John Lind had tried to tell them this, but it took them forty-two years to get the message.** Then they went overboard and decided that if fruits prevent scurvy, then meat causes scurvy!

Some of the scurvy stories are remarkable and pathetic. The prospectors in the Yukon gold rush often died unnecessarily from Vitamin C deficiency—scurvy. They would sicken near the end of the winter. Having an abiding faith in raw potatoes as a cure for scurvy, and they do indeed contain Vitamin C, the sick prospector's comrades would often go to heroic lengths to bring potatoes from great distances for their friend. Usually they were too late. The tragedy was that caribou milk, which was generally available, would have saved them with little effort. Also, they were walking on tons of Vitamin C in the form of tundra grass, moss and lichens.

---

* That's right, the Irish. The Norsemen didn't show up until 160 years later.

** What is it about doctors? Does medicine in every age attract students with the most immobile minds?

Although physicians of the 19th century had made up their minds that lime juice was *the* specific for scurvy, it constantly failed when put to severe test.* Sir George Nares returned from a polar expedition in 1876 to report that in spite of lime juice they had had much scurvy and death. The doctors, clinging to their lime juice theory, said that absence of sunlight and *lack of amusement* had nullified the good effects of the marvelous juice!

Nansen returned from a very successful expedition with no illness among his men in 1876.[31] They had no sunlight and no entertainment. They did not take lime juice but lived on walrus meat and fat. Although Nansen's books were best sellers, undoubtedly read by thousands of doctors of the period, *doctors continued to pontificate on meat causing scurvy.***

The doctors and scientists never ran out of excuses for lime juice. Why, it was asked, did it appear to work better in the 18th century than the 19th? It took a while to explain that one, but eventually they did. They announced triumphantly that the meaning of "lime" had changed. In the 18th century the juice was made from lemons called limes. Now it's made from limes called lemons.

This travesty of scientific thought was repeated over and over again. In the early 20th century, the explorer Scott failed on two expeditions because of scurvy. He followed the advice of the leading physicians of the day and carried lime juice. The first expedition was a disaster, and the second one was worse. All of them, including Scott, died of scurvy only ten miles from the final provision depot. Not one of them would have died if the doctors had only heeded the simple advice of Nansen about eating fresh meat and advised Scott accordingly.

---

* As there was no refrigeration, the juice would rapidly lose Vitamin C potency.

** Even if this book becomes a best seller, because of the typical M.D. mentality, it will have little or no effect on the contemporary practice of nutritional medicine.

I'm not trying to convince you to eat nothing but meat. The brilliant work of Stefansson is presented to demonstrate some of the inaccurate and harmful beliefs of present-day nutrition. You *could* live on nothing but raw meat, you *could* live well on nothing but raw milk, and you *could live* well on nothing but raw vegetables (especially green grass).

The ancients of Egypt were a powerful race. They performed incredible intellectual and physical feats. We still can't figure out how they built the pyramids. They were basically omnivorous. They consumed their vegetables *raw* and got their meat from temple sacrifices.

In the 17th century, Indians of the Northwest Territory lived a vigorous life exclusively on meat. French explorers of that period were dying of scurvy.[32] They were in what is now the state of Minnesota. One of the men made friends with an Indian. The Indian liked him and told him that he would cure his scurvy if the Frenchman promised not to tell the other members of the expedition. After the Frenchman promised, the Indian killed a buffalo, cut out the adrenal gland and had him eat it raw. He became well almost immediately.

The Indians had never heard of Vitamin C, so they didn't know that Vitamin C would cure scurvy, and they did not know that the adrenal gland contains the highest concentration of Vitamin C in the body of animals. But the Indians knew that if they ate the whole animal, intestines, liver, brain, bone marrow, heart, and especially the adrenal glands, *and ate it raw,* they would remain healthy and vigorous.

The people of Lichtenstein, a tiny country adjoinf¬g Switzerland, lived almost exclusively on milk and milk products for centuries. *Many of them lived to be one hundred to one hundred-fifty years of age.* [33]

The Samburu tribe of northern Kenya continues to baffle the cholesterol-fat alarmists.[34] They drink nothing but milk for three days and then eat nothing but meat for one day. The sequence may vary, but in general, there are three milk days to one meat day. Pasteurization is unknown to them. The milk is cultured, similar to yogurt.

They eat *four hundred grams* of fat per day. The average American, with his hardened arteries, eats a meager *eighty grams* of fat per day. The Samburu warrior, by tribal tradition, is bound from age fourteen to an *exclusive diet of milk* and meat for twenty years. No vegetable products are eaten except for some tree bark tea.

The Samburu's cousins to the south, the Masai,* drink an average of seven quarts of very rich milk per day. Their diet is 60% saturated fat. When you consider that the average warrior weighs only one hundred thirty-five pounds, that's a lot of milk.

It is true that the Masai also drink the blood of animals. But contrary to popular belief, blood is not a routine part of their diet. Blood is drawn only when milk is in short supply as an emergency procedure.

Mann and co-workers studied these tribes exhaustively.[35] They found remarkably little heart disease, consistently normal blood pressure,** no obesity, and a complete absence of rheumatoid arthritis, degenerative arthritis, and gout.

What about cholesterol? The average African child had a cholesterol value of 138. The average American child, 202. With increase in age, the native cholesterol values went *down* and the American values went *up*. Beyond the age of fifty-five, the mean cholesterol value of the African natives was *122*. The American mean cholesterol for men was *234*.

---

* As you know, they are both of Nilo-Hamitic extraction.
** The mean blood pressure at age sixty was 125/76.

In his conclusions, Mann did not equivocate, "(The studies) show no support for the contention that a large intake of dairy fat and meat necessarily causes either hypercholesterolemia or coronary heart disease... the hypothesis relating saturated animal fat to the causation of hypercholesterolemia and cardiovascular disease remains dubious. (We) favor the conclusion that diet fat is not responsible for coronary disease."

Dr. Kurt Biss, et al, confirmed Dr. Mann's work in 1971.[36] They performed autopsies on the natives and found, in spite of their enormous cholesterol and animal protein intake, that they were essentially free of artherosclerosis including their heart arteries. They also found that "...the Masai are virtually free from cholesterol gallstones."

The American Heart Association and many nutrition professors in prestigious universities have gone way out on a limb concerning fat and cholesterol in our diet. They have recommended a shift to less milk, eggs, meat—what they mistakenly call "saturated" fats—to a diet containing more margarine, fish, and vegetable oils. They are committed. They must continue to support their completely untenable and nutritionally disastrous position or admit that they have made a terrible mistake.*

The American Heart Association, the principle promoter of the fat-cholesterol theory of atherosclerosis, is now going after the children and recommending low-cholesterol diets for 3 *year olds*. But the American Academy of Pediatrics is striking back. They point out that cholesterol is vital in growing children for the formation of bile salts, hormones, and nerve tissue. *There is no population of children that has been raised on such a radical diet.* Yet the American Heart Association assures America's mothers

---

*Can you imagine those professors admitting that they have been giving the wrong advice?

that "There appear to be no demonstrated major hazards involved" if the kids follow the AHA's radical diet plan.*

But they go on to admit that "...several epidemiologic studies... have failed to observe significant correlations among dietary fat, serum cholesterol concentrations and coronary heart disease rates." You can find studies to prove either position depending on whether you study the Masai tribesmen, the Ni-Hon-San of Japan, or business executives at Western Electric.**

In one study by Pearce and Dayton that the AHA did *not* mention, it was found that eight years on a low cholesterol, high unsaturated fat diet caused a twofold increase in *cancer*.[37] One actually needs only 2% of calories in the form of polyunsaturated fat. A slice of good bread laden with butter should do it. But the AHA is recommending a drastic increase to *20% unsaturated fat.*

For whichever reason, political or scientific, the Food and Drug Administration refused to be sucked into endorsing reckless and unproven dietary recommendations to the American people. Doctor Herbert Ley, Commissioner of the FDA, said, "The scientific correlation between ...(fat) and arteriosclerosis is an extremely tenuous one. Although there is a great deal of publicity, there is very little fact that clearly links the ingestion of fat in one form or another with heart disease."

But eight years later another branch of the government did the FDA in. On January 14, 1977, the Senate Select Committee on Nutrition and Human Needs, known as the McGovern Committee, issued a report advising the American people to change their diet. They recom-

---

* Fortunately, a low cholesterol diet is boring and so children won't stay on it. Just ask a Pritikin graduate how long he stayed with the diet.

** Wouldn't it make more sense just to go back and study our grandparents? They ate plenty of lard, butter, eggs and milk, but coronary heart disease was rare.

mended that the consumer reduce his saturated fat and cholesterol consumption by a whopping 40%.*

The Senators, unqualified in science, were given the hard sell by Dr. Gio Gori of the National Cancer Institute. He said that fat was a major factor in cancer, and they bought it. Doctor Jean Mayer of Harvard endorsed the report, but not everyone was taken in.

Doctor Thomas Jukes of the University of California, said, "Senator McGovern's Committee on 'nutrition and human needs' has issued a preposterous report on 'dietary goals' which calls for governmental action to implement the prejudices of the writers... I don't think they know what they're talking about."

Nutrition professor George Briggs seconded it, "Meat, milk and eggs are among our best foods and we are a healthier nation because we have such good supplies. We need to consume more, not less."

The report had a pronounced effect on various government departments and health-oriented foundations. The Department of Agriculture went so far as to issue a regulation *requiring* schools to make low-fat milk available to students (See page 35 about the unhealthy properties of low-fat and skim milk.) The National Cancer Institute joined the gaggle honking for a holy war on whole milk, meat, and eggs.

The worst case of cholesterol phobia on record must be that of Doctor Walter W. Sackett, Jr., of Miami, Florida. Dr. Sackett, a prominent physician and member of the Florida legislature was quoted in the National Enquirer as saying, "Milk is more deadly than cigarettes because the cholesterol it contains contributes to a million deaths a year in the United States." He tells his patients that he "... would rather see them smoke a cigarette than drink

---

* Why would they do this when the dietary cholesterol intake, in the past eighty years, has only increased 1%?[38]

one glass of milk... this is murder ...cholesterol kills you... surely and ever so slowly."*

Patricia Hausman, in her anti-milk, anti-meat book, *Jack Sprat's Legacy,* said, "When the last quarter of the 20th century is recorded in history books, the American Heart Association, the Senate Select Committee on Nutrition... and other organizations that have advocated less meat or less meat fat, may well look like revolutionaries." They may also look like fools.**

There are numbers of ways that you can eat raw animal protein other than raw milk, raw eggs, oysters, and clams.*** Most people have heard of the seasoned raw hamburger dish called Steak Tartar, although few have tried it. It's delicious. The Italians have a wonderful dish called Carpacio. It's very thinly sliced raw beef with a white sauce—magnifique. Kibe, a North African dish, is made from raw lamb. Not bad, but not as good as Steak Tartar. The Japanese, and remarkably, a rapidly increasing number of Americans, eat raw fish called Sushi. Once you try it, you'll be hooked.

Want to live to be a hundred? Eat mostly raw animal protein, and you may make it.****

Rather than follow a diet from a government report based on screwed up arithmetic, you are better off listening to Stefansson, the explorer, and Dr. Mann of the Samburu studies. They dealt in reality, not supposition

---

* Sackett admitted to smoking three packs of cigarettes a day.

** Go ahead and read her book, and then decide for yourself. C.S.P.I., 1775 "S" Street, NW, Washington, D.C., 20009.

*** Did you know that raw oysters and clams are actually alive when you eat them? So are fertilized eggs. The Japanese eat a live prawn called Odori. It tickles your mouth as it jumps around. It doesn't want to be eaten.

**** If industrial pollutants, an 18-wheeler, or modern medicine don't get you first.

and politics. You don't have to eat like a rabbit to maintain good health. You can eat like a tiger and do just as well, maybe better.

Find out which dairy in your community feeds its cows the best diet, and then drink their milk—unpasteurized. If you can't find any unprocessed cow milk, look for goat milk. For some illogical reason, some states, such as Rhode Island, allow the sale of unpasteurized goat milk and outlaw raw cow milk. Others, like Florida, look the other way concerning the sale of raw goat milk.

Udderly Unique

Goats are different from most farm animals. They are more tuned to the good life. They romp a lot and have a sense of humor. Like pigs, a goat will be clean and orderly if given a chance.* Goats are very passionate. If you don't think so, just visit a goat farm during the mating season.**

You probably never wanted to know that the West African dwarf goat's milk is remarkably rich in protein as is the Oregonian pygmy goat. With goats, quality comes in small packages. Worldwide, the dwarf strains produce the best milk.

Goat's milk is not bad. I was going to write a separate chapter on goat's milk, but research convinced me that goat's milk is really not that different from cow's milk. If both are in the raw state, goat's milk and cow's milk are equally digestible.[39] If you can't drink one, it isn't likely that you can digest the other. If you want to drink goat's milk, it's okay. Just be sure the milk is raw and certified. It is rich and delicious.

Health food oriented people generally consider goat's milk to be more digestible and more nutritious than cow's milk. They are probably wrong on both counts. When com-

---

* A goat will not grunt in his gazebo.
** It's downright embarassing.

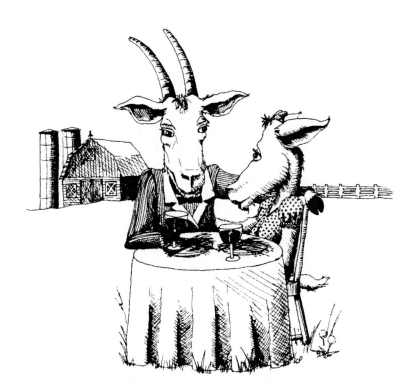

Goats are Neat. Cows don't Care.

paring goat's milk to cow's milk, as far as digestibilty is concerned, the comparison is generally between raw goat's
milk and *pasteurized* cow's milk. When both are raw, there
appears to be little or no difference in digestibility.[40]

Pasteurization is the basic difference that makes
cow's milk appear less digestible than goat's milk. If you
pasteurize goat's milk, you're right back to a processed,
de-natured product.*

The professors say there is no difference, but the curd
of goat's milk is smaller, and many people who cannot
drink cow's milk (pasteurized) are able to drink goat's milk.

Goat milk devotees claim that goat milk fat is more
digestible because the fat globules are smaller. On the average, goat milk fat globules are smaller, but if this contention were true, then homogenized cow milk fat with
its very tiny globules should be more digestible. Experimental evidence doesn't support this contention.[41]

There are some areas where cow's milk is clearly superior to goat's milk. Goat's milk is deficient in Vitamin
B1, Vitamin B12, and especially folic acid. "Goat milk
anemia"[42] has been reported in children fed exclusively
on goat's milk.[43] It responds quickly to folic acid treatment. Another study, reported in the Yearbook of the
American Goat Society,[44] attempts to refute these findings. They reported that children fed goat's milk developed better than those fed cow's milk. But these were not
infants living exclusively on goat's milk. Babies should
have human breast milk. Horse's milk would be the second choice; raw cow's milk properly diluted is third.

The contention that goat's milk is less likely to cause
allergic reactions than cow's milk also is not borne out by
the scientific literature. A study done by Johns Hopkins University[45] showed no significant differences in the allergy potential of the two milks. If you are allergic to *raw* cow's
milk, you will probably be allergic to *raw* goat's milk.

---

* If you don't understand that, you have missed the whole point of
this book. Start over.

Goat's milk is okay, but in my opinion, not worth the extra expense except in special circumstances. And remember, goats are subject to the same diseases as cows. Check to see if the operation is clean. Probably more important, ask the farmer if *his* family drinks the milk. If they do, you can be reasonably certain that the milk is clean.

But there is one great advantage to goat's milk—availability. In many states where raw cow's milk is not available, raw goat's milk can be obtained if you just make the effort. Ask at your local health food store. Many state legislatures seem to look the other way regarding raw goat's milk.

We need to put in a plug for fried food. Frying per se has never been proven to be any worse than boiling, baking, or broiling.* The important factors in frying are:

1) The type of fat used.

2) The temperature at which the food is cooked. Extremely high temperatures not only destroy vitamins, fat, and protein values, but convert some foods to atherogenic and/or carcinogenic substances.

3) The length of time the food is cooked.

Most doctors, if asked whether fried foods are unhealthy, would probably say "yes." One envisions grease pouring into the liver, the gallbladder groaning in complaint, and the bowels in a discontented and spastic upheaval. No one knows why fried food is bad. Everybody just knows it's bad. While doctors feel confident that they are on sound ground in making the assertion that fried

---

* This doesn't mean that we recommend the french fries at your local finger-lickin'-good fast food chain. They are boiled in coconut, peanut, or palm oil.

food is probably bad, most of them eat fried food like everybody else.

You will probably be as surprised as I was to find practically nothing in a search of the literature on the effect of fried foods on the digestion. The one article on the subject refutes the old medical prejudice, against fried foods.

Boggess and Ivy did their frying experiment with potatoes. They concluded that pan-fried potatoes were more easily digested than French fried.*

Dr. Frank Howard Richardson, commenting on the prejudice against frying,[46] said, "There is a widely held belief, cherished by physicians and laity alike, to the effect that fried foods are harmful in general and that they are particularly harmful for children. An analysis... clearly demonstrates that it is not documented with scientific proof or with any proof at all for that matter. Rather, it is merely a repetition and reiteration in many different forms of this unproved old unscientific prejudice."

Food that is pan-fried in butter or one of the edible oils such as sunflower, linseed, and olive oil or safflower oil, is no worse than any other cooked food. In fact, Boggess in his experiment found that fried potatoes were more digestible than boiled potatoes.

Please Pass the Grass

America's golf courses grow enough nutritious food to supply a large proportion of our nutrient needs. Cows aren't very smart, but when given a chance, they eat better than most Americans.

Green grass contains twenty-three times as much Vitamin A as carrots, twenty-two times as much Vitamin B2

---

*French fry is a misnomer. Boiling in grease is not the French way. The French pan-fry or saute. McDonald's and Col. Sanders "french fry."

as lettuce, nine times more thiamin than green leafy vegetables, and fourteen times more Vitamin C than citrus
fruits! The humble blade also contains niacin, Vitamin E,
and probably nutrients not yet discovered. It's also
packed with minerals and enzymes. Professor Johnston-
Wallace declared, "About five pounds of dried tender
grass would supply enough vitamins to last a man an entire year."

You don't like green grass? That's the point of this
dissertation on grass. Milk from cows fed green grass
converts this perfect vegetable to a palatable form for
man. Green grass milk is the closest thing to a perfect
food. However, most commercial milk contains *none* of
the green grass factors because the cows from these mass
production milk factories *never see* green grass.

Randleigh Farms[47] did an experiment that should
convince you that your children should drink only raw
milk from green grass fed cows. Two barns housed eleven
cows each. The one group received the same feed as the
other except green hay and fresh green wastes were
added. They produced normal calves year after year.

The group not receiving the green supplements,
while producing an equal quantity of milk the first year,
rapidly dropped off in milk production the second year.
Many stopped breeding, and by the third year, the group
receiving no green feed produced only one normal calf.

John P. O'Neil, M.D., said in 1948, "The overcoming
of disease cannot be accomplished until soil, agriculture,
medical science, and veterinary science are amalga-
mated.[48] Dr. O'Neill pointed out that the foods we eat are
no better than the soils they come from, and this includes
animals as well as plants. If a cow is raised on poor soil
and therefore gets poor grass, she will produce nutritionally inferior milk. If a race horse is raised on poor grass,
he will not become a winner. I would not have believed
the importance of that if it wasn't for the story told by Dr.
O'Neill at a meeting of the certified milk producers.

One of the largest racing stables in the country had for decades produced brood mares and stallions of the highest quality. Their horses were always big winners and made a fortune for their owners. These magnificent animals, known for their robust health and speed, were raised in the heart of the blue grass country of Kentucky.

In 1933, after years of successful racing, things began to go wrong. They lost money that year. In seven years the stable was in ruins. In 1941 they had sixty thoroughbreds racing, but most of them seemed to be going backward. The stallions weren't racing, and the mares weren't producing.* The few foals dropped were either stillborn or deformed.

What a disaster! The "experts" said that the blood lines had "run out" and advised them to sell the animals for dog food and start over. But the manager of the stable was knowledgeable in agricultural science and knew that the horses could only be as good as the soil and grass that raised them. He suggested to the owner that he call in soil chemists before turning his expensive and carefully bred animals into shoe leather.

He took the manager's advice, and the horses were saved from the glue factory. It wasn't the horses. It was the soil. It contained practically no minerals or other nutritional elements. Even the worms, essential to good soil maintenance, were gone. In only two years, after growing well-fertilized crops with cattle and plowing under the green crops for rejuvenation of the soil, the worms returned. By 1945, *with the same stock of mares and stallions,* they were in third place in winnings in the United States.

What affects horses also affects cows. If the milk you are drinking is not from cows fed the very best grass from rich soil, you are not getting your money's worth in nutrition from the milk. This has been proven beyond a doubt.[49] Put garbage in and you get garbage out as inferior milk.

---

*The stallions weren't chasing the mares either.

Dr. Francis Pottenger reported on a study of cats fed cooked meat.[49] One of the cats gave birth to six kittens. She ate two of them on the first day, three died of diarrhea on the third day, and the last one died the next day. Dr. Pottenger said that milk supply was usually inadequate, the mother showed little inclination to feed them, and the kittens had narrow, poorly developed faces. This was the pattern when the mother had been fed on heated food such as cooked meat and pasteurized milk.

Dr. Pottenger illustrated how this carries over into human maternal nutrition. A family was studied in which the mother's diet had varied considerably with different children. The first born infant was the lucky one. The mother was living on a farm drinking not less than two quarts of raw milk every day produced by a cow fed fresh cut alfalfa. The child was well developed and healthy.

The sister came along at a time when the mother was consuming a deficient diet. She had the narrow face and poor skeletal development seen in Pottenger's cats. He summarized, "...skeletal development is... directly in proportion to the amount of green feed entering into the milk fed the infants."

So, remember that green grass is an incredibly good food for human consumption. If you ever get caught in a famine situation, just eat the grass—you'll do okay.

REFERENCES

1. *The Fat of the Land*, Macmillan, 1956, pp. XXXVII.

2. *In the Shadow of Man*. New York, Houghton Mifflin, 1971.

3. Olduvai Gorge, Vol. 3, Oxford, Cambridge University Press, 1971.

4. Martin, Natural History, 76:32-38 (1967).

5. Abrams, Journal of Applied Nutrition, Vol. 31, #1 & 2, 1979.

6. Harner, Natural History, 86:46-51 (1977).

7. Johanson, Science, 203:321 (1979).

8. Abrams, Jr., App. Nut. 31 #1 and 2, 1979.

9. J.D. Science, Vol. 5, #3, pp. 297.

10. Br. J. Nut., 16:476-74 (1962).

11. Nutrition Program News, July / August (1973).

12. Nutrition Reviews, 37:142-144 (1979).

13. Enig., et al, Fed. Proc. 37:2215 (1978).

14. JAMA, 189:655-59 (1964).

15. N. England Journal Medicine, 98:317 (1978).

16. Abrams, J. App. Nutr., Vol. 32 #2, pp. 53-87.

17. Ibid., p. 65.

18. Journal of Applied Nutrition vol. 31 #1, 1979.

19. Abrams, J. App. Nut., 32, #2 (1980).

20. Your Body is Your Best Doctor, Page & Abrams, Keats Publ., Conn. (1974).

21. *The Cultural Dimension of the Human Adventure,* MacMillan, New York, 1979.

22. Ibid.

23. *TheFat of the Land,* Stefansson, Macmillan, 1956, pp.91.

24. Nature, 252:158 (1974).

25. Winkler, et al, Amer. Journal of Med., Vol. 46, February 1969, pp. 297.

26. Resurrection, et al, Nutrition (2586-2591).

27. *Adventures in Diet,* Harper's Magazine, November/December 1935, January 1936.

28. Personal conversation with Icelander, Eggert Edwald, Reykjevik, Iceland, Summer 1983.

29. *The Fat of the Land,* Stefansson, Macmillan, 1956.

30. Op. cit.

31. Op. cit.

32. *The Value of Good Foods & Vitamins,* Dr. Lowell A. Erf, History of Randleigh Farms.

33. Op. cit.

34. Cardiovascular Disease of the Masai.

35. Op. cit.

36. N.E.J. Medicine, Vol. 284, #13, pp. 694, April 1971.

37. JAMA, December 28, 1970, Vol. 214, #13.

38. Jenness, Journal Dairy Science, Vol. 63, #10, 1980.

39. Ibid.

40. Trout, Journal Dairy Science, 31:627, 1948.

41. Parkash, Dairy Science Abstr., 30:67, 1968.

42. Davidson, J. Pediatrics, 90:590, 1977.

43. Mack, Yearbook of American Goat Society, 1953.

44. Ibid.

45. Gamble, U.S. Dept. Agriculture Tech. Bulletin, 671, 1939.

46. The Journal of Pediatrics, February 1944.

47. History of Randleigh Farms.

48. Speech at annual banquet of Certified Milk Industry, Waukeska, Wisconsin, June 20, 1948.

49. Elvehjen, Journal Dairy Science, Vol. 17 (12), pp. 763;

Chapter XIII

ICE CREAM

"So delectable as to be near a sin."
— Anonymous, probably God.

You need the scoop on ice cream.

If you are an ice cream freak like me, watching the manufacture of ice cream at Alta-Dena Dairy is almost a religious experience. The temple is the storage area where rich, luscious, creamy, natural (raw cream), gorgeous ice cream is stacked three stories high!* Alta-Dena ice cream is the only raw milk, raw cream, completely natural ice cream available in the entire United States on a commercial basis. That tells you a lot about the status of our food supply.

Nero, the Emperor of Rome in the first century, B.C., was an ice cream nut. He would have royal runners fetch snow from the mountains. The kitchen would cover it with honey, fruit, or wine. Nero loved his ice mixture so much that he made it illegal for everyone but himself.**

In the 13th century, Marco Polo proved that the Chinese were ahead of us in practically everything. He brought back an ice cream formula from the Orient.

King Charles the First was also an ice cream freak. He issued a 17th century royal decree to his cook that he must not divulge his ice cream recipe to the peasants.***

---

*It is 20 degrees below zero in the temple, so I didn't stay in church very long.

** No one paid any attention.

*** It was too good for them, and besides, Charles was a selfish bastard.

George Washington was crazy about the frozen delight. He kept two silver pots just for his ice cream. Dolly Madison served it at the White House.

Alta-Dena ice cream isn't cheap. Neither is Hagen-Das, Copenhagen, Mathis, or Shiloh Farms, other top quality brands. But with ice cream, cost and quality don't always go together. A survey in Chicago, for example, rated one of the lowest priced ice creams as the best and the most expensive as "awful." This was a flavor test and had nothing to do with nutritional value. When eating ice cream, one doesn't usually think about nutrition, but you can have ice cream that is both nutritious and delicious. Most ice creams are delicious and poisonous.

The first commercial ice cream was marketed in 1851 in Baltimore. The producers at that time didn't know how to make "modern" ice cream. They thought all you needed was raw milk, fresh eggs, cream, butter, and natural flavors. Today a typical commercial ice "cream" contains skim milk, two kinds of sugar, our favorite waste product-whey, mono- and diglycerides, polysorbate 80,* guar gum, chemical flavors such as vanillin (pronounced van' ah lin),** chemical colors, and carrageenin. That's only the beginning. I'll come back to additives after I tell you about the Alice in Wonderland called "Standard of Identity."

With most processed foods, regulations require that the processor tell you on the label what the product contains. Granted, many of these regulations are vague enough, and although they don't have to tell you what has been done to the product, they must at least say on

---

*I don't have the slightest idea.

**It's made from wood pulp treated with sulfuric acid. It only costs about ten cents a gallon more to use real vanilla which comes from a tropical orchid. Don't want extract of wood pulp instead of vanilla? Don't complain because you will get piperohal instead. If you ask Orkin, they'll tell you piperohal is a lice exterminator.

the label what has been added. Not the pasteurized-ho-mogenized milk boys.

Milk and milk products have a "Standard of Identity." I put that in caps and quotes because it's a magical term the bureaucrats of the Agriculture Department invented to allow the milk industry to get away with murder—or at least nutritional mayhem.

They don't *have* to tell you what's in the milk you feed your kids because the government regulators have given milk producers special dispensation. They have said, essentially, that everyone recognizes milk and milk products; we trust the milk producers; milk is milk and so they don't have to tell us what they are putting in it as long as they heat it before selling it.

Hard to believe? Ask the National Dairy Council, Rosemont, Illinois 60018 to send you a copy of publication B300-1-1978 entitled *Newer Knowledge of Milk.* Table three on page fourteen is very revealing. They don't have to tell you *anything* about the nutritional content of pasteurized milk or ice cream. They can add chemical coloring, emulsifiers, stabilizers, chemical flavors, and "nutritive sweeteners" (that's sugar to you and me), and *they don't have to inform you on the label.** The same brand may even be different from one week to the next.

That's the magic of "Standard of Identity," a confusing term meaning simply: License to deceive.

Grandmother never realized it, but ice cream is held together electrically. There are only *eighteen tablespoons* of liquid in a full gallon of ice cream. It's mostly air, oil, and ice crystals suspended in water.** Air, oil, and water don't mix very well. It's the negative electrical charges that keep everything in suspension and give us that sinfully delicious mix.

---

* Presumably, they could put WD-40 in their products if they wanted to.

** The poorer the ice cream the more air and ice crystals. What's cheaper than air and ice?

The main ingredient in ice cream, besides air, is milk fat. There's only one reason the ice cream manufacturers use milk fat. It's not legal to call it ice cream if you don't use milk fat. With the current national phobia about cholesterol and animal fat this may change. Non-dairy ice cream, like non-dairy everything else made from coconut oil and peanut oil, would seem inevitable. It's already standard in England.

In fact, as the refinement of our foods continues, don't be surprised to find "ice cream" that requires no refrigeration. Leave it in a box on your pantry shelf for a year. When you are ready for some of the noble glop, add water, mix it in your blender, and pop it into your freezer.*

We told you about using the human mouth as a disposal system back in our junk milk chapter. The ice cream makers do it too. Water pollution laws since 1960 forced the cheese companies to find a new way to dispose of whey.** The human gullet has proven ideal, and it's a cheap way to increase the milk solids in the ice cream to the legal minimum limit. Dr. Philip G. Keeney, Department of Dairy Science, Penn State University, commented, "Nobody uses whey for positive reasons. They use it because it's cheap and it's allowed."[1]

Whey has a metallic flavor that a buzzard wouldn't like, but enough sugar and artificial flavor will cover anything. Dr. Keeney concluded, "In a way, ice cream has become the sewage treatment plant of the cheese industry."[3]

Now we come to the *bad* part.

When you order a banana split at your neighborhood ice cream parlor, you may get vanilla flavored ice cream, chocolate, and strawberry. But you will probably get iperonal (a lice killer) for vanilla, amylphenyl acetate for chocolate, and a solvent called benzyl acetate for

---

*Why fool around? A half-ton cow must eat thirty pounds of feed and filter 2,500 gallons of blood through her udder to make one lousy quart of cream.[2]

** It smothers fish.

strawberry. The toppings will probably be aldehyde C-17 for cherry, ethyl acetate for pineapple,* rutyraldehyde for nut flavor, and a paint solvent called amyl acetate for that great banana flavor. It's all economics. Aldehyde C-17 costs seven cents per gallon of ice cream. Real cherries cost thirty-five cents a gallon.

There are over a *thousand* different chemicals used in commercial ice cream. How about those beautiful colors added to ice cream to make your Little One's birthday a truly memorable event? You will get tartrazine (yellow) to upset his little stomach, dissamine red 6B for red, and indiotine for blue. He can also be poisoned with amaranth, ponceau2R, and titanium dioxide.** Coal tar dyes are the major source of artificial coloring. Many of them are known to be potent cancer-causing agents.

A single ice cream may contain as many as fifty-fiue chemical ingredients. If you really go el cheapo, you might get refiner's syrup as the "nutritive sweetener." Refiner's syrup is the last liquid product of the sugar refining process. It has been described by technicians in the field as "practically inedible."

You need a good emulsifier to make ice cream. It gives it a characteristic stiffness and richness. Grandmother, not being wise in economics and knowing nothing about chemicals, used fresh eggs from the hen house. Today they use diethylglycol, an anti-freeze, and polyoxyethylene which is suspected of causing cancer. They also use polysorbate 65. It deceives you into thinking that the ice cream has a high cream content. As a thickener you may find dioctyl sodium sulfosuccinate which is a chemical used in medicine as a stool softener.***

One of the most common additives to ice cream is carageenin. When this chemical is added to water and

---

* Ethyl acetate vapors cause lung, liver, and heart damage.

** Who knows? Maybe he had a titanium deficiency anyway.

*** Just in case you needed it.

fed to guinea pigs, they develop ulcers. Some scientists think it may cause ulcerative colitis in humans.

Commercial ice cream is loaded with sugar. Sugar causes diabetes, and according to Dr. Norman Kretchner of Stanford University, sugar is a major cause of athero-sclerosis. A person with hypoglycemia (low blood sugar) may faint or have a convulsion from eating sugar-laden commercial ice cream. The convulsions may be from the sugar, or the chemicals, or both.

We could tell you about the additive CMC causing tumors and polysorbate-80 causing premature death in experimental animals, but I guess you get the message: If you want to go on an eskimo pie in the sky trip, eat commercial ice cream.

Something else you should know. Unlike milk, there are no federal standards setting the maximum number of bacteria to be allowed in ice cream. As we pointed out in Chapter IV, *pasteurized* ice cream has been a not infrequent source of food poisoning epidemics.

They really get away with murder when they sell you "reworked" ice cream. "Reworked" is a euphemism for covering up stale ice cream and selling it as fresh. They just throw it back with the fresh, add more chemicals, and presto—America's fun food.

If you like chocolate, please raise your hand.* The best way to disguise the poor quality of reworked ice cream is to add a lot of chocolate. There's not much good news about chocolate and a lot of bad. If you don't want to be turned off on chocolate, skip to page 250.

The following information on chocolate comes from the newsletter of Tom Cooper, M.D. of Atlanta, Georgia. As I can't improve upon it, I am repeating it here:

"Almost everyone with a weight problem has a chocolate problem... Since I have a hard time resisting

---

*I knew you did. Everybody likes chocolate.

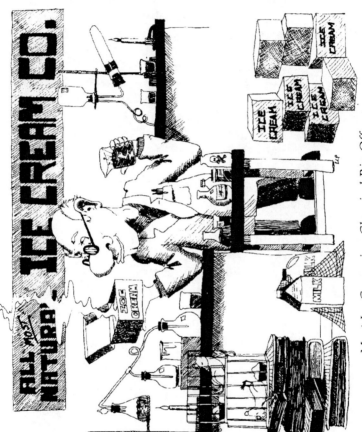

Most Ice Cream is a Chemical Rip-Off.

chocolate I decided to see if there was anything about it that would turn me off. I struck paydirt in the first reference book I consulted and in a Food and Drug Administration policy guideline reference publication.

It seems that candy bars don't grow on trees after all! Over half of the chocolate we consume comes from cocoa trees found in West Africa in countries like Ghana, Nigeria, Ivory Coast, and Cameroon. The cocoa tree grows in a lush tropical environment and has a number of fungi and insects that are enemies to this plant. It is necessary to spray the trees with a number of control chemicals, including organic and potentially toxic fungicides that could remain in small amounts in the harvested cocoa beans.

The cocoa trees produce a certain number of seed pods each year. These pods are harvested, and the cocoa beans are removed manually by natives. They are then spread out on the jungle floor and allowed to ferment (a nice way to say rot) for five to six days in the jungle heat and humidity. There is nothing to keep insects and small animals from nesting and feeding among the beans while they are exposed to the elements. It is common to find animal droppings, dead insects, and animal hairs in this fermenting collection of cocoa beans.

After they have stayed like this for the required period of time, they are packed in jute or plastic bags and stored in harbor warehouses until it is time to load them into the holds of ships for transportation to this country. In the warehouses and the ship holds they are again subjected to the ravages of resident rodents and insects. The cocoa bean is a rich source of fats and carbohydrates and is relished by both kinds of pests.

The resulting mixture of cocoa beans, insect fragments, rodent droppings, leaves, and rat hairs is unloaded in this country and is taken to one or another of the various chocolate processing factories. A conscientious effort is made by these companies to remove as many of these contaminants as they possibly can, but the thousands of tons of raw material processed each month make this a virtual impossibility.

To quote the FDA manual, 'The action levels are set because it is not now possible, and never has been possible, to grow in open fields, harvest, and process crops that are totally free of natural defects.' Translate natural defects into hairs, insect fragments, and animal waste. There is, and I know you will be comforted to know this, a level at which the FDA will seize a product and not let it be sold.

If 100 grams (about three ounces) of chocolate exceeds an average of 60 microscopic insect fragments or one rodent hair when six similar samples are analyzed, or if any one sample contains more than 90 insect fragments or three rodent hairs, then this sample will be rejected by the FDA. I suppose this means that if there are only 59 insect fragments, or only one rodent hair per 100 grams then we are alright!

Animal waste is normally the color of chocolate and cannot be tested for with any great accuracy. The cooking process destroys almost all the germs, so I guess this means that it is reasonably healthy. Nobody is hurt by this contamination, since the hairs and insect fragments are partly protein, but the aesthetic aspect of chocolate with all this possible filth mixed with it has made me less likely to eat it. I am afraid that when I bite into a candy bar, the crunch may not come from peanuts, but from something else."[4]

A word of caution on sherbets. Avoid them as you would soggy cigarette butts. This "light, cool, summer delight" is strictly bottom of the line. Sherbets have very little milk solid. The milk solids are replaced by a heavy dose of additives and sugar. There's over a pound of sugar in a gallon of sherbet.

The National Dairy Council,[5] whose job is to inform the American people about dairy products, says, "Rigid government standards assure consumers of (ice cream's) purity, healthfulness, and high quality."*

So, belly up to the ice cream bar and order an Anti-Freeze Frappe', Sorbitam Soda, Lice Killer Cooler, Paint Solvent Sundae, a Terasodium Pyrophosphate Split, or a Red Dye Delight—ummm yummie.

Eating Germs for Good Health
(Yogurt, Kefir, and Koumiss)

Raw milk is good food, but cultured raw milk is even better. Many people who cannot drink pasteurized milk can drink raw milk. But some can't even drink that. They just can't handle the lactose. This would be very frustrating in trying to treat patients with milk therapy. But, fortunately, we have cultured ("fermented") milk to work with.

These cultured products, yogurt, kefir, and koumiss, are pre-digested.** The fat, sugar, and protein has been partially broken down making them digestible for practically everyone.

A large percentage of Negroes and other dark-skinned races cannot tolerate milk pasteurized or raw. But many tribes in Africa practically live on cultured milk from their herds.

It is claimed that people who rely heavily on cultured milk in their diet live longer. In some areas of Rus-

---

* Rigid government standards? Purity? High quality? *Healthfulness?* They even recommend it as a "breakfast surprise." Makes you want to throw up.

** There are other cultured milks such as Keldermilk from Norway and Skyr from Iceland. Basically, they are about the same.

sia, where large amounts of koumiss* are consumed, there are a large number of people who live to be a hundred or more. Nikita Khrushchev, the former dictator of Russia, said that three times as many people lived to be one hundred years old in his country than in the United States.** Benet reported in 1971[6] that in one small Black Sea village there were one hundred eighty people over ninety-one years old. These people were rarely sick, and atherosclerosis was uncommon. They drank a lot of cultured milk.

Yogurt consumption has skyrocketed in the United States in recent years and is expected to be a billion dollar business by 1986.[7] Kefir, a liquid product with different and even better bacteria than yogurt, is coming on fast. It's consistency is about halfway between yogurt and buttermilk. That makes it just right for the American palate, sort of like a milkshake, and I predict that it will eventually overtake yogurt in consumption. Koumiss will never make it in this country although it's probably the best of the lot. (Closer to human milk). It contains five times more Vitamin C than cow milk.***

The trouble with yogurt in this country is the same as the rest of our food. When the product caught on, the big food producers moved in with their sugared, pasteurized phony yogurt. People have a vague conception that yogurt is good for them, a "health food." But, when polled, most hadn't the vaguest notion why. Most polled didn't know that billions of live, friendly bacteria make yogurt yogurt. These bacteria not only predigest the fat, sugar, and protein. They also "crowd out" lethal bacteria in the gut. Perhaps even more important, these microorganisms *manufacture their own antibiotics* to destroy disease-causing germs.

---

* Pronounced 'ku meece'. It's made from horse milk.

** He didn't make it. Too much vodka.

*** But Americans just won't drink horse milk.

One of these good germs is called lactic-acid strep.*
It suppresses spoilage germs, and that's why African natives can use it without refrigeration.

As most consumers aren't aware of the importance
of these bacteria in their yogurt, the manufacturers can
get away with cultures with a low count or *absolutely no
bacteria*. This is really pathetic because they think they
are getting a longer shelf life by pasteurizing out all of
the friendly bacteria, where actually the opposite is
true.**

I told you about the therapeutic effectiveness of raw
milk. With yogurt and kefir you can multiply that effectiveness by at least two, maybe more. Fermented milk
therapy is big in Russia. There are over fifty sanitaria in
the Soviet Union using cultured milk therapy.*** For a serious disease the patient is fed a quart and a half of cultured milk, usually koumiss, daily.[8]

Elias Metchnifkoff, a Russian scientist who worked
with Louis Pasteur, was the first distinguished scientist**** to claim that cultured milk has great therapeutic
value. Seventy years later he is being taken seriously in
this country. A host of new and effective antibiotics have
been isolated from the bacteria of cultured milk,[9] lacto-
bacillin, bulgarian, lactobrevin, and many others. Many
deadly organisms are controlled by this new breed of antibiotics from fermented milk.

Milk will lower cholesterol, but yogurt and kefir will
do it better. A unique "anti-cholesteremic milk factor"
has been discovered in fermented milk.[10] What this factor is remains a mystery.

---

* Not the kind that causes strep throat.

** When they rape the product of all the good bacteria, they
should make them call it Nogurt rather than Yogurt.

*** For koumiss production, the Russians are milking *250,000
horses*. It's not enough to fill the demand.

**** He had won the Nobel Prize in medicine in 1908.

Want to improve your sex life?* We don't guarantee you anything, but consider the story of Dr. Edward Spieker of Munich, Germany. He came to the United States in 1937 to promote a product unknown to the American people—yoghurt.** He had eaten yogurt all of his life.

He was accompanied by Countess Alma von Blucher, "a friend of the family." The year before he had had his second child by his second wife. He was seventy-two years old. He still had hair on his head *and needed no glasses.****

There are three reasons why yogurt, kefir, and koumiss prolong life. They protect against infection because of the built-in antibodies, they are protective against hardening of the arteries, and there is a potent anti-cancer effect.[11]

There is surprisingly little research on this important aspect of cultured milks. A check with the American Cancer Society on this exciting avenue of research brought the following response: "   ."****

The original research on the anti-cancer effect of cultured milks was done twenty years ago.[12] Work at the Sloan-Kettering Institute for Cancer Research has confirmed and enlarged on the original studies. They found that Lactobacillus acidophilus "possessed definite anti-tumor activity.*****

Added to all the above advantages is the fact that yogurt, kefir, and koumiss are more nutritious than milk. They are much higher in B vitamin content and Vitamin C, and the protein is the very highest quality available for human consumption.

---

* Who doesn't?

** That's the way they used to spell it.

*** We have been unable to determine his present place of residence. If alive, he's only 120.

**** I wrote to them twice.

***** Maybe the American Cancer Society doesn't speak to Sloan-Kettering either.

Perhaps the most remarkable quality of cultured milks is their ability to protect against radiation injury. Dr. Tomic-Karovic exposed guinea pigs to X-ray. He found that those receiving cultured milk did not have abnormalities in their offspring. Those not protected by the milk had birth defects. Would it not be wise for every expectant mother to add kefir or yogurt to her diet?"*

REFERENCES

1. Science '81, Terry Dunkle, July / August.

2. Ibid.

3. Ibid.

4. Food and Food Encyclopedia, Considine, 1982, Van Nostrand Co., NYC. FDA Compliance Policy Guides Manual.

5. National Dairy Council, B103, 1979.

6. The New York Times Magazine, December 26,1971.

7. Milk Industry Foundation, Milk Facts, 1978.

8. Cheese and Fermented Milk Foods.

9. Shahani, J. Dairy Science, 1979, 62:1685.

10. Mann, 1977, Atherosclerosis 26:335.

11. Op. cit.

12. Bogdanov, 1962, Abstr. VIII Int. Cancer Cong., pp. 364.

*Make sure it's yogurt and not nogurt.

APPENDIX I

State	Raw Milk	Raw Certified Milk
1. Alabama	May not be sold.	May not be sold.
2. Alaska	No data.	No data.
3. Arizona	May be sold.	May be sold.
4. Arkansas	Sold at farm.	No law.
5. California	May be sold.	May be sold.
6. Colorado	May not be sold.	No law.
7. Connecticut	May not be sold.	May be sold.
8. Delaware	May not be sold.	May not besold.
9. District of Columbia	May not be sold.	May not be sold.
10. Florida	May not be sold.	May not besold.
11. Georgia	May not be sold.	May be sold.
12. Hawaii	May not be sold.	No law.
13. Idaho	May be sold.	May besold.
14. Illinois	Sold at farm..	No law.
15. Indiana	May not be sold.	May not be sold.
16. Iowa	Sold at farm.	Sold at farm.
17. Kansas	Sold at farm.	Sold at farm.
18. Kentucky	May not be sold.	May not be sold.
19. Louisiana	May not be sold.	No law.
20. Maine	May not be sold.	No law.
21. Maryland	May not be sold.	May not besold.
22. Massachusetts	No law.	No law.
23. Michigan	Sold at farm.	No law.
24. Minnesota	Sold at farm.	Sold at farm.
25. Mississippi	May not be sold.	May not besold.
26. Missouri	Sold at fann.	No law.
27. Montana	May be sold.	No law.
28. Nebraska	Sold at farm.	No law.
29. Nevada	May not be sold.	May be sold.
30. New Hampshire	May be sold.	No law.
31. New Jersey	May not be sold.	May be sold.
32. New Mexico	Sold at farmL.	No law.
33. New York	May be sold.	May be sold.
34. North Carolina	May not be sold.	May not besold.

State	Raw Milk	Raw Certified Milk
35. North Dakota	May be sold.	No law.
36. Ohio (*)	May not be sold.	Allowed. (*)
37. Oklahoma	Sold at farm.	No law.
38. Oregon	May be sold.	May be sold.
39. Pennsylvania (**)	Allowed. (**)	Allowed. (**)
40. Rhode Island (***)	Allow Raw Goat's Milk Only	
41. South Carolina	Sold at farm.	May not be sold.
42. South Dakota	May not be sold.	No law.
43. Tennessee	May not be sold.	May not be sold.
44. Texas	Sold at farm.	No law.
45. Utah	May be sold.	May be sold.
46. Vermont	No law.	No law.
47. Virginia	May not be sold.	May not be sold.
48. Washington	May be sold.	May be sold.
49. West Virginia	May not be sold.	May not be sold.
50. Wisconsin	May not be sold.	May not be sold.
51. Wyoming	May be sold.	No law.

---

* Ohio—Allow if farm was in business before 1965.

** Pennsylvania—Not sold in eating establishments.

*** Rhode Island—All milk except goat's milk is pasteurized.

APPENDIX II

Household Test for Contaminated Milk

Dr. J. Howard Brown of Johns Hopkins University described a method of testing milk for "dirt," as he called it. That's a euphemism for cow manure.

Spore-forming bacteria are germs with a protective shell around them, like a walnut. They never come directly from the milk and so, if found, are positive evidence of contamination of the milk from manure, stall dust, dirty utensils, or dirty milking attendants. *They are not killed by pasteurization* because of their protective shells.

One of these organisms found in manure produces gas if the oxygen supply is cut off. Any housewife can do the test to prove the presence of this gas-forming bacteria.* It may seem like a lot of fuss, but a few gurgling milk cartons may make you think twice about drinking "pasteurized" milk. Raw certified milk will rarely, if ever, be positive for these fecal bacteria.

Take a large kettle in which a quart of milk may stand with the water coming up to within an inch of the top.** Start with cool water. Open the carton, but cover the opening lightly with a piece of aluminum foil. To prevent bumping, place a rack under the carton. A few large hair pins will do.

Bring the water to a vigorous boil. Then remove the carton from the boiling water and set aside to cool, leaving the aluminum foil loosely on top.

---

* Clostridium welchii.
** This is easier to do with old-fashioned milk bottles.

After the carton has cooled enough to be handled, press the foil around the top of the container and place the carton upside down in a clean container of water with the top of the milk carton resting on the bottom. The water should come half-way up the side of the milk carton.

Put your experiment in a warm area of the house and examine daily. If gas-forming fecal bacteria are present, in a few days the bacteria will have blown most of the milk out of the bottle.*

---

*You will be glad you didn't drink it.

APPENDIX III
Definition of Certified Milk

The following description and definition is reproduced verbatim from the September, 1938 issue of Certified Milk Magazine:

"Rules and regulations for the production of certified milk are laid down by a national organization of physicians, The American Association of Medical Milk Commissions. Each certified farm is supervised by a local Medical Milk Commission, members of which are appointed by the local medical society, and each Medical Milk Commission is a member of the national organization.

Certified milk is the product of cows that are in perfect health. The milk of each is tested for healthfulness before each milking. The slightest indication of anything wrong with a cow results in her instant withdrawal from the certified herd to which she is not restored until again in perfect health.

Cows used to produce certified milk are steadily cared for by experienced veterinarians who regularly examine and test them. These cows are housed in well lighted, well ventilated barns kept always scrupulously clean. Before each milking, each cow's flanks and udder are brushed, washed, and cleansed so no outside dirt may get into the milk.

Only men in perfect health may work about cows used to produce certified milk, These men are kept in perfect health by steady attention of physicians and regular health tests and examinations. If anything is found wrong with a man's health, he cannot afterward go near the certified dairy until he is pronounced entirely well.

Men who work about certified dairies are required to keep themselves at all times scrupulously clean. They wear clean white gloves, their hands are regularly manicured and frequently washed, and all their personal habits are under constant supervision.

Cows used for production of certified milk are fed most carefully balanced and measured rations so that certified milk may at all times be of uniformly high quality.

Certified milk, as soon as it is taken from the cows, is cooled, bottled, sealed and kept in refrigeration until used.

These precautions, plus frequent and regular bacterial tests, insure a milk of dependable purity, cleanliness, flavor and freshness. Only such milk may bear the designation Certified Milk."

APPENDIX IV

A Suggested Baby Feeding Formula
(Natural, raw Certified Milk)

1. Human milk = 20 calories per ounce.
   Regular formula (excluding premature) = 20 calories per ounce.

2. Certified Milk corrected to 20 calories per ounce may be prepared as follows:

   1) Boil all nursing bottles, nipples, and measuring cups in water 20 minutes. Then, refrigerate them, including water.

   2) Remove cap from a one quart bottle of Certified Milk which has been well shaken. Place cap on a clean paper towel or other clean surface.

   3) Pour off 6 ounces of Certified Milk for other use, i.e., drink it.

   4) Pour into the residual 26 ounces of Certified Milk one ounce White Karo Syrup.

   5) Add 5 ounces of the boiled, then REFRIGERATED, water.

   6) Replace a clean cap and shake well. The bottle is sterile and ideal for storage.

7) At each feeding, shake well and pour the necessary
    amount of milk into sterile bottle. Warm to room
    temperature under a hot water tap.

TO SOFTEN STOOLS, you may add: First, one to
two ounces dark Karo; second, one to two ounces
B'rer Rabbit Molasses. If two ounces of any of the
above must be added, omit one ounce water, and it
will still fit into a sterile one quart bottle. The calorie count will be only slightly higher.

This formula is recommended for babies of
normal birth weight to 15+ pounds or 6+
months old, then continue using Certified
Milk, undiluted.

For further information, call your doctor, or
R.L. Mathis Certified Dairy: (404) 289-1433.

APPENDIX V

"Oleomargarine Tax Repeal." Hearings before the committee on agriculture, House of Representatives, 80th Congress, 2nd Session, U.S. Government Printing Office, Washington, D.C., 1948.

Oleomargarine Tax Repeal

Mr. Andresen. You are, in fact, representing Best Foods?

Dr. Deuel. In fact, representing what I know about the nutritional value of vegetable fats. I am not representing Best Foods. I was asked by Best Foods to be here.

Mr. Andresen. And compensated by them for your appearance?

Dr. Deuel. I am compensated to the extent that my railroad fare from Chicago here and back to Cincinnati is paid for by them.

Mr. Andresen. I can say to you, doctor, I have enjoyed your statement and the answers to my questions. There has been no question in my mind as to the value of one product as against another, but the controversy here is color, yellow, and you have refrained in your statement from mentioning the color yellow. All that I want is oleo and margarine sold for what it is, and not as an imitator of butter, which is the usual case. That is all.

The Chairman. Mr. Murray.

Mr. Murray. I would like to ask questions of the gentleman, but he has a great deal of background. There are certain statements that the gentleman has made that, to me, are very disturbing. No. 1. The gentleman is trying to come to the conclusion that a vegetable oil is equal to an animal fat, but by his own admission he had not proven that by his own experiments. The oleo margarine you have used, you say, contained around 15 percent dairy products; is that right?

Dr. Deuel. I think about 13 percent.

Mr. Murray. Well, according to the Oleo Institute, it is 15.6 percent. In answer to the gentleman from Minnesota, you also said that you implemented the ration by adding casein, which is another dairy product. Your test does not show it and I have never seen an experiment yet that proved that a vegetable oil was equal to an animal fat and none of your experiments prove that. Am I right or wrong?

Dr. Deuel. In the first place, I want to call your attention to the fact that I am speaking solely about the fat. We are talking about fats here. You get no casein whatsoever from butter except what is in the skimmed milk portion that is present. You get just as much in margarine. I am not saying that you can eat oleomargarine and eat nothing else and get along. You cannot. You will die just as quickly if you eat oleomargarine as you will with butter, if you have nothing else. You must have protein, you must have calories, which you cannot get from those. You must have minerals, you must have the fat soluble vitamins, the water soluble vitamins. I am simply claiming that those substances which we need, which we ordinarily look to the fat for, are as completely in margarine, fortified margarine, as they are in butter. That is all I am saying.

Mr Murray. Well, what you are saying, then, is that the vegetable oil if implemented by casein and skimmed milk —is then equal to butter. I am not admitting it, but that is your position?

Dr. Deuel. May I add one more statement? If one attempts to get the things like excellent casein from butter, solely from butter, then, you are in a position where you will get into a terrific condition nutritionally. You will be short on your protein and I would advise a person who is short and wants to get a well-rounded diet to take whole milk, because that is where you get your casein, that is where you get your salts. It is not in butterfat.

Mr. Murray. Dried skimmed milk has 1 percent butterfat in it, so any experiment of yours that you have seen does not prove that the vegetable oil is as good as the animal fat. I am not talking dairy or nondairy, just from an experimental standpoint. If your contention is right, then, you have to say that this Milnot, which is composed of 94 percent dairy product and 6 percent vegetable oil is just as good as evaporated natural milk; is that right?

Dr. Deuel. I have never investigated Milnot and I know nothing about it whatsoever.

Mr. Murray. Well, on the thesis that a vegetable oil is equal to an animal fat, there is no reason why that is not just as good, if it is doctored up the same way?

Dr. Deuel. I can only testify on experiments which I have done myself and which I know about. I cannot give any testimony on Milnot.

Mr. Murray. But your conclusion is that a vegetable oil is equal to an animal fat even though you use dairy products to prove it.

Dr. Deuel. If you want to interpret it that way, that is all right, but I cannot interpret it that way.

Mr. Murray. I do not know any other interpretation to make.

Dr. Deuel. I can only interpret on the basis of what I have done. I know nothing about Milnot and I have never read the label so I do not know what the product is.

Mr. Murray. But in principle, if a vegetable oil is equal to an animal fat, it surely does not spoil it by putting more skimmed milk in it?

Dr. Deuel. I have never written that and I do not choose to say that now.

Mr. Murray. How about this oleo cheese? The only difference between that and natural cheese is that this was made out of soybean oil instead of cottonseed oil. I am afraid I would be tempted to tell all the subsidies cotton has and I would not to get the blood pressure up that way. Here is a cheese made out of soybean oil, some 31/2 percent. If your conclusions are correct, then, that is just as good as natural cheese. I am not saying your conclusions are correct, but if you have proven that a vegetable oil is equal to an animal fat, that is just as good as a piece of natural cheese.

Dr. Deuel. Well, they have certain types of cheese that are very excellent and very well thought of, made out of goat's milk, have they not?

Mr. Murray. Sure.

Dr. Deuel. They probably have them made out of different kinds of milk.

Mr. Murray. This is soybean oil cheese I am talking about, oleo cheese.

Dr. Deuel. Does that contain skimmed milk?

Mr. Murray. Yes.

Mr. Murray. Then, according to your contention, it might be just as good as this cheese.

Dr. Deuel. I imagine it would, but I have no experiments on such cheese.

Mr. Murray. Here is No. 3. A bottle of milk made down here in the dairy department.

Dr. Deuel. Made by a cow, is it not?

Mr. Murray. It has 4 percent soybean oil in it. It has been homogenized, and, according to you, if a vegetable oil is equal to an animal fat that is just as good as a quart of natural milk. I am not admitting it, but I am just submitting it to you to show you how far down the road we are going.

Your experiment, or no experiment, has yet ever proven that a vegetable oil is equal to an animal fat because you have never had an experiment that you did not have to lean on the old cow when you were running the experiment.

As far as the oleo trust is concerned—or whatever it is —I am getting sick of all the high-power propaganda that they put into this thing because they are misleading the people. I hope you do not subscribe to that Chicago experiment and base your reputation on that Chicago experiment with those children for 2 years' time.

If you read that article, what did it say? How much percentage of fat did the children get as vegetable oil?

Dr. Deuel. They got what they would normally take. I have it right here.

Mr. Murray. How much of it came from animal fat? Just read the experiment. It will show you how unfair that experiment is. I was sorry to have you subscribe to it because I have a high respect for all scientists. I was surprised because your fellow scientist was here 3 years ago and told us that oleo was just as good as butter, and it only had 9,000 international units. Then they found out that butter had from 15,000 to 27,000, and now they come back and say it is just as good and has 15,000. I do not know what they will say the next time they come in here for a hearing, if they ever have to come back again.

I do not know whether the testimony was right that time or this time. I do not know whether that testimony is right or whether yours is right.

Dr. Deuel. It states in here that the margarine substituted approximately 65 to 70 percent of the total fat calories.

Mr. Murray. In other words, they get a third of their fat as animal fat in the ration, and therefore they run a wonderful experiment.

Dr. Deuel. Does it say that the other 30 percent was animal fat? It might just as well have been vegetable fat. Many vegetables contain appreciable amounts of —

Mr. Murray. Do you mean to tell me those children went 2 years without any milk?

Dr. Deuel. I do not know.

Mr. Murray. Why were they not honest about it and publish the facts if they wanted to run an experiment based on common, ordinary horse sense.

Dr. Deuel. I would not choose to dispute a plan of experiment set up by Prof. Anton Carlson. He is the most honest and sincere individual that I know in American science.

Mr. Murray. He might be honest, but he might be like some of the rest of us and make mistakes. I heard a gentleman within 30 minutes telling people they ought to use oleomargarine for cooking when it only has 3,300 calories, and you can buy a pound of lard for 23 cents which has 22 percent more calories in it than oleomargarine and the oleo costs 70 percent more money per pound.

I am not saying anything against the man personally, but that experiment surely would not stand on its own feet if those children had milk which includes butterfat.

Now, what difference does it make if they drink enough milk? What good is the experiment?

Dr. Deuel. That is exactly what I have been saying. If we diverted more of our milk to drink as whole milk we would be a whole lot better off than if we tried to give the milk to the pigs and make the fat into butter.

I am not against whole milk. I am for whole milk, and I am for a larger consumption of whole milk by our children and by our adults.

Mr. Murray. But you have to have a skim-milk cow.

Dr. Deuel. No. I am saying: Drink whole milk. Butterfat is a good fat, but it is not superior to the vegetable oils. It will not do things that the vegetable oils will not do.

Mr. Murray. As a scientist, can you tell people they should use oleomargarine in comparison to lard, talking about the low-income groups, when lard has 22 percent more calories?

Dr. Deuel. Would you prefer to eat lard to oleomargarine?

Mr. Murray. For cooking, sure.

Dr. Deuel. On your table?

Mr. Murray. You did not say that.

Dr. Deuel. I said cooking and table use.

Mr. Murray. As far as I am concerned, I would rather eat lard than oleo. Then I would not be kidding myself. This is a serious matter to me. Just because I come from a State that happens to have a few cows, they all try to put it on that basis.

I was in Wisconsin when the first vitamin A or fat soluble A experiment was run. I am not a chemist, but I can read what they say in the book. What gets me is that now we come in here with the Best Foods, or whatever the name of that company is, and have a scientific man come in and tell this committee that they have an experiment anywhere in this world—they have never had one yet— that shows that a vegetable oil is equal to an animal fat. It has not been done, and they have never run an experiment yet that did not have to lean up on the old dairy cow to get part of the products going into the experiment.

I defy anybody to dispute that statement of fact in the record.

APPENDIX VI

Biblical and Other Ancient References to Meat and Fat.

Genesis IV, 2-5:

Isaiah XXV, 6 (King James): "And in this mountain shall the Lord of hosts make unto all people a feast of fat things, a feast of wines on the lees, of fat things full of marrow."[1]

Ancient Icelandic poem: "There (in paradise) the feast will be set clear wine, fat and marrow."[2]

Lev. III, 3, 9, 16,17

Lev. VII, 3, 23

"And Abel was a keeper of sheep, but Cain was a tiller of the ground."

"And in process of time it came to pass, that Cain brought of the fruit of the ground an offering unto the Lord."

"And Abel, he also brought of the firstlings of his flock and of the fat thereof. And the Lord had respect unto Abel and to his offering."

"But unto Cain and to his offering he had not respect."

Genesis XLIX, 20: "Out of Asher his bread shall be fat, and he shall yield royal dainties."

Nehemiah VIII, 9: "Then he said unto them, Go your way, eat the fat, and drink the sweet."

Genesis XIV, 17-18: "And Pharaoh said unto Joseph— Take your father and your households, and come unto me: and I will give you the good of the land of Egypt, and ye shall eat the fat of the land."

The Illiad, Book XII: "Verily our kings that rule Libya be so inglorious men, they that eat fat sheep, and drink the choice wine honey-sweet."

REFERENCES

1. Holy Bible.
2. *The Fat of the Land*, Stefansson, Macmillan, 1956.

ABOUT THE AUTHOR

Dr. William Campbell Douglass is a fourth generation physician. His family has been serving the state of Georgia since 1850. He is a graduate of the University of Rochester, New York; the University of Miami School of Medicine; and the United States Naval School of Aviation and Space Medicine. Dr. Douglass travels the world giving lectures, doing radio and TV talk shows and gathering health information that is not covered by our press. He has spent a lifetime searching out the inexpensive, natural cures that really do "make things right"—including extensive on-site research into the revolutionary hydrogen peroxide and ultra-violet blood irradiation therapies. Dr. Douglass was voted Doctor of the Year in 1985 by the National Health Federation, and was a founding member and state president of the Florida American College of Emergency Physicians.

INDEX

About Doctor William Campbell Douglass II

Dr. Douglass reveals medical truths, and deceptions, often at risk of being labeled heretical. He is consumed by a passion for living a long healthy life, and wants his readers to share that passion. Their health and well-being comes first. He is anti-dogmatic, and unwavering in his dedication to improve the quality of life of his readers. He has been called "the conscience of modern medicine," a "medical maverick," and has been voted "Doctor of the Year" by the National Health Federation. His medical experiences are far reaching-from battling malaria in Central America - to fighting deadly epidemics at his own health clinic in Africa - to flying with U.S. Navy crews as a flight surgeon - to working for 10 years in emergency medicine here in the States. These learning experiences, not to mention his keen storytelling ability and wit, make Dr. Douglass' newsletters (Daily Dose and Real Health) and books uniquely interesting and fun to read. He shares his no-frills, no-bull approach to health care, often amazing his readers by telling them to ignore many widely-hyped good-health practices (like staying away from red meat, avoiding coffee, and eating like a bird), and start living again by eating REAL food, taking some inexpensive supplements, and doing the pleasurable things that make life livable. Readers get all this, plus they learn how to burn fat, prevent cancer, boost libido, and so much more. And, Dr. Douglass is not afraid to challenge the latest studies that come out, and share the real story with his readers. Dr. William C. Douglass has led a colorful, rebellious, and crusading life. Not many physicians would dare put their professional reputations on the line as many times as this courageous healer has. A vocal opponent of "business-as-usual" medicine, Dr. Douglass has championed patients' rights and physician commitment to wellness throughout his career. This dedicated physician has repeatedly gone far beyond the call of duty in his work to spread the truth about alternative therapies. For a full year, he endured economic and physical hardship to work with physicians at the Pasteur Institute in St Petersburg, Russia, where advanced research on photoluminescence was being conducted. Dr. Douglass comes from a distinguished family of physicians. He is the fourth generation Douglass to practice medicine, and his son is also a physician. Dr. Douglass graduated from the University of Rochester, the Miami School of Medicine, and the Naval School of Aviation and Space Medicine.

You want to protect those you love from the health dangers the authorities aren't telling you about, and learn the incredible cures that they've scorned and ignored?
Subscribe to the free Daily Dose updates "...the straight scoop about health, medicine, and politics." by sending an e-mail to real_sub@agoramail.net with the word "subscribe" in the subject line.

Dr. William Campbell Douglass'
Real Health:

Had Enough?

Enough turkey burgers and sprouts?

Enough forcing gallons of water down your throat?

Enough exercising until you can barely breathe?

Before you give up everything just because "everyone" says it's healthy...

Learn the facts from Dr. William Campbell Douglass, medicine's most acclaimed myth-buster. In every issue of Dr. Douglass' Real Health newsletter, you'll learn shocking truths about "junk medicine" and how to stay healthy while eating eggs, meat and other foods you love.

With the tips you'll receive from Real Health, you'll see your doctor less, spend a lot less money and be happier and healthier while you're at it. The road to Real Health is actually easier, cheaper and more pleasant than you dared to dream.

Subscribe to Real Health today by calling 1-800-981-7162 or visit the Real Health web site at www.realhealthnews.com.
Use promotional code : DRHBDZZZ

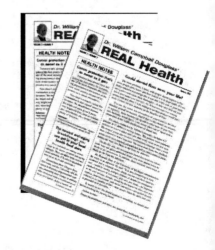

If you knew of a procedure that could save thousands, maybe millions, of people dying from AIDS, cancer, and other dreaded killers....

Would you cover it up?

It's unthinkable that what could be the best solution ever to stopping the world's killer diseases is being ignored, scorned, and rejected. But that is exactly what's happening right now.

The procedure is called "photoluminescence". It's a thoroughly tested, proven therapy that uses the healing power of the light to perform almost miraculous cures.

This remarkable treatment works its incredible cures by stimulating the body's own immune responses. That's why it cures so many ailments--and why it's been especially effective against AIDS! Yet, 50 years ago, it virtually disappeared from the halls of medicine.

Why has this incredible cure been ignored by the medical authorities of this country? You'll find the shocking answer here in the pages of this new edition of Into the Light. Now available with the blood irradiation Instrument Diagram and a complete set of instructions for building your own "Treatment Device". Also includes details on how to use this unique medical instrument.

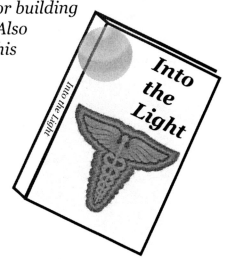

Rhino Publishing S.A.
www.rhinopublish.com

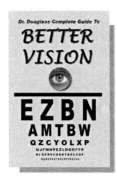

Dr. Douglass' Complete Guide to Better Vision

A report about eyesight and what can be done to improve it naturally. But I've also included information about how the eye works, brief descriptions of various common eye conditions, traditional remedies to eye problems, and a few simple suggestions that may help you maintain your eyesight for years to come.
-William Campbell Douglass II, MD

The Hypertension Report.
Say Good Bye to High Blood Pressure.

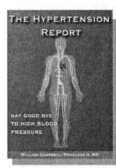

An estimated 50 million Americans have high blood pressure. Often called the "silent killer" because it may not cause symptoms until the patient has suffered serious damage to the arterial system. Diet, exercise, potassium supplements chelation therapy and practically anything but drugs is the way to go and alternatives are discussed in this report.

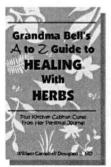

Grandma Bell's A To Z Guide To Healing With Herbs.

This book is all about - coming home. What I once believed to be old wives' tales - stories long destroyed by the new world of science - actually proved to be the best treatment for many of the common ailments you and I suffer through. So I put a few of them together in this book with the sincere hope that Grandma Bell's wisdom will help you recover your common sense, and take responsibility for your own health. -William Campbell Douglass II, MD

Prostate Problems:
Safe, Simple, Effective Relief for Men over 50.

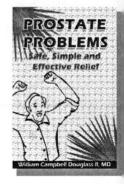

Don't be frightened into surgery or drugs you may not need. First, get the facts about prostate problems... know all your options, so you can make the best decisions. This fully documented report explains the dangers of conventional treatments, and gives you alternatives that could save you more than just money!

Color me Healthy
The Healing Powers of Colors

"He's crazy!"
"He's got to be a quack!"
"Who gave this guy his medical license?"
"He's a nut case!"

In case you're wondering, those are the reactions you'll probably get if you show your doctor this report. I know the idea of healing many common ailments simply by exposing them to colored light sounds far-fetched, but when you see the evidence, you'll agree that color is truly an amazing medical breakthrough.

When I first heard the stories, I reacted much the same way. But the evidence so convinced me, that I had to try color therapy in my practice. My results were truly amazing.

-William Campbell Douglass II, MD

Order your complete set of Roscolene filters (choice of 3 sizes) to be used with the "Color Me Healthy" therapy. The eleven Roscolene filters are # 809, 810, 818, 826, 828, 832, 859, 861, 866, 871, and 877. The filters come with protective separator sheets between each filter. The color names and the Roscolene filter(s) used to produce that particular color, are printed on a card included with the filters and a set of instructions on how to fit them to a lamp.

Rhino Publishing
www.rhinopublish.com

What Is Going on Here?

Peroxides are supposed to be bad for you. Free radicals and all that. But now we hear that hydrogen peroxide is good for us. Hydrogen peroxide will put extra oxygen in your blood. There's no doubt about that. Hydrogen peroxide costs pennies. So if you can get oxygen into the blood cheaply and safely, maybe cancer (which doesn't like oxygen), emphysema, AIDS, and many other terrible diseases can be treated effectively. Intravenous hydrogen peroxide rapidly relieves allergic reactions, influenza symptoms, and acute viral infections.

No one expects to live forever. But we would all like to have a George Burns finish. The prospect of finishing life in a nursing home after abandoning your tricycle in the mobile home park is not appealing. Then comes the loss of control of vital functions the ultimate humiliation. Is life supposed to be from tricycle to tricycle and diaper to diaper? You come into this world crying, but do you have to leave crying? I don't believe you do. And you won't either after you see the evidence. Sounds too good to be true, doesn't it? Read on and decide for yourself.

-William Campbell Douglass II, MD

Rhino Publishing S.A.
www.rhinopublish.com

HYDROGEN PEROXIDE

Medical Miracle

H_2O_2

Eat Your Cholesterol!

Eat Meat, Drink Milk, Spread The Butter- And Live Longer!
How to Live off the Fat of the Land and Feel Great.

Americans are being saturated with anti-cholesterol propaganda. If you watch very much television, you're probably one of the millions of Americans who now has a terminal case of cholesterol phobia. The propaganda is relentless and is often designed to produce fear and loathing of this worst of all food contaminants. You never hear the food propagandists bragging about their product being fluoride-free or aluminum-free, two of our truly serious food-additive problems. But cholesterol, an essential nutrient, not proven to be harmful in any quantity, is constantly pilloried as a menace to your health. If you don't use corn oil, Fleischmann's margarine, and Egg Beaters, you're going straight to atherosclerosis hell with stroke, heart attack, and premature aging -- and so are your kids. Never feel guilty about what you eat again! Dr. Douglass shows you why red meat, eggs, and dairy products aren't the dietary demons we're told they are. But beware: This scientifically sound report goes against all the "common wisdom" about the foods you should eat. Read with an open mind.

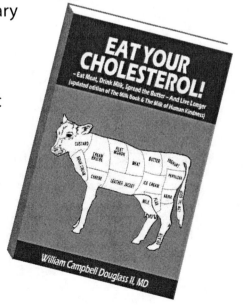

Rhino Publishing, S.A.
www.rhinopublish.com

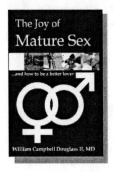

The Joy of Mature Sex
and How to Be a Better Lover

Humans are very confused about what makes good sex. But I believe humans have more to offer each other than this total licentiousness common among animals. We're talking about mature sex. The kind of sex that made this country great.

Stop Aging or Slow the Process
How Exercise With Oxygen Therapy
(EWOT) Can Help

EWOT (pronounced ee-watt) stands for Exercise With Oxygen Therapy. This method of prolonging your life is so simple and you can do it at home at a minimal cost. When your cells don't get enough oxygen, they degenerate and die and so you degenerate and die. It's as simple as that.

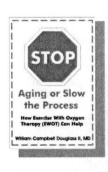

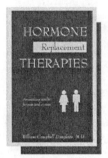

Hormone Replacement Therapies:
Astonishing Results For Men And Women

It is accurate to say that when the endocrine glands start to fail, you start to die. We are facing a sea change in longevity and health in the elderly. Now, with the proper supplemental hormones, we can slow the aging process and, in many cases, reverse some of the signs and symptoms of aging.

Add 10 Years to Your Life
With some "best of" Dr. Douglass' writings.

To add ten years to your life, you need to have the right attitude about health and an understanding of the health industry and what it's feeding you. Following the established line on many health issues could make you very sick or worse! Achieve dynamic health with this collection of some of the "best of" Dr. Douglass' newsletters.

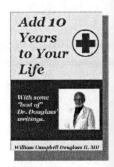

How did AIDS become one of the Greatest Biological Disasters in the History of Mankind?

GET THE FACTS

AIDS and BIOLOGICAL WARFARE covers the history of plagues from the past to today's global confrontation with AIDS, the Prince of Plagues. Completely documented *AIDS and BIOLOGICAL WARFARE* helps you make your own decisions about how to survive in a world ravaged by this horrible plague.

You will learn that AIDS is not a naturally occuring disease process as you have been led to believe, but a man-made biological nightmare that has been unleashed and is now threatening the very existence of human life on the planet.

There is a smokescreen of misinformation clouding the AIDS issue. Now, for the first time, learn the truth about the nature of the crisis our planet faces: its origin -- how AIDS is really transmited and alternatives for treatment. Find out what they are not telling you about AIDS and Biological Warfare, and how to protect yourself and your loved ones. AIDS is a serious problem worldwide, but it is no longer the major threat. You need to know the whole story. To protect yourself, you must know the truth about biological warfare.

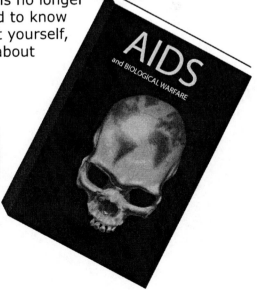

Rhino Publishing S.A.
www.rhinopublish.com

PAINFUL DILEMMA

Are we fighting the wrong war?

We are spending millions on the war against drugs while we
should be fighting the war against pain with those drugs!

As you will read in this book, the war on drugs was lost a long time ago and,
when it comes to the war against pain, pain is winning! An article in USA Today
(11/20/02) reveals that dying patients are not getting relief from pain. It seems
the doctors are torn between fear of the government, certainly justified, and a
clinging to old and out dated ideas about pain, which is NOT justified.

A group called Last Acts, a coalition of health-care groups, has released a very
discouraging study of all 50 states that nearly half of the 1.6 million Americans
living in nursing homes suffer from untreated pain. They said that life was being
extended but it amounted to little more than "extended pain and suffering."

This book offers insight into the history of pain treatment and the current failed
philosophies of contemporary medicine. Plus it describes some of today's most
advanced treatments for alleviating certain kinds of pain. This book is not another
"self-help" book touting home remedies; rather, Painful Dilemma: Patients in
Pain -- People in Prison, takes a hard look at where we've gone wrong and what
we (you) can do to help a loved one who is living with chronic pain.

The second half of this book is a must read if you value your freedom. We now
have the ridiculous and tragic situation of people
in pain living in a government-created hell by
restriction of narcotics and people in prison for
trying to bring pain relief by the selling of
narcotics to the suffering. The end result of the
"war on drugs" has been to create the greatest
and most destructive cartel in history, so great,
in fact, that the drug Mafia now controls most
of the world economy.

PAINFUL DILEMMA
PATIENTS IN PAIN
PEOPLE IN PRISON

Rhino Publishing S.A.
www.rhinopublish.com

Live the Adventure!

Why would anyone in their right mind put everything they own in storage and move to Russia, of all places?! But when maverick physician Bill Douglass left a profitable medical practice in a peaceful mountaintop town to pursue "pure medical truth".... none of us who know him well was really surprised.

After All, anyone who's braved the outermost reaches of darkest Africa, the mean streets of Johannesburg and New York, and even a trip to Washington to testify before the Senate, wouldn't bat and eye at ducking behind the Iron Curtain for a little medical reconnaissance!

Enjoy this imaginative, funny, dedicated man's tales of wonder and woe as he treks through a year in St. Petersburg, working on a cure for the world's killer diseases. We promise --

YOU WON'T BE BORED!

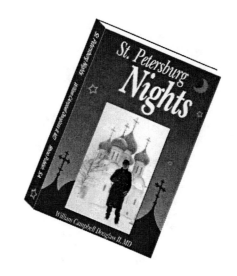

Rhino Publishing S.A.
www.rhinopublish.com

THE SMOKER'S PARADOX
THE HEALTH BENEFITS OF TOBACCO!

The benefits of smoking tobacco have been common knowledge for centuries. From sharpening mental acuity to maintaining optimal weight, the relatively small risks of smoking have always been outweighed by the substantial improvement to mental and physical health. Hysterical attacks on tobacco notwithstanding, smokers always weigh the good against the bad and puff away or quit according to their personal preferences. Now the same anti-tobacco enterprise that has spent billions demonizing the pleasure of smoking is providing additional reasons to smoke. Alzheimer's, Parkinson's, Tourette's Syndrome, even schizophrenia and cocaine addiction are disorders that are alleviated by tobacco. Add in the still inconclusive indication that tobacco helps to prevent colon and prostate cancer and the endorsement for smoking tobacco by the medical establishment is good news for smokers and non-smokers alike. Of course the revelation that tobacco is good for you is ruined by the pharmaceutical industry's plan to substitute the natural and relatively inexpensive tobacco plant with their overpriced and ineffective nicotine substitutions. Still, when all is said and done, the positive revelations regarding tobacco are very good reasons indeed to keep lighting those cigars - but only 4 a day!

Rhino Publishing, S.A
www.rhinopublish.com

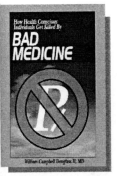

Bad Medicine
How Individuals Get Killed By Bad Medicine.

Do you really need that new prescription or that overnight stay in the hospital? In this report, Dr. Douglass reveals the common medical practices and misconceptions endangering your health. Best of all, he tells you the pointed (but very revealing!) questions your doctor prays you never ask. Interesting medical facts about popular remedies are revealed.

Dangerous Legal Drugs
The Poisons in Your Medicine Chest.

If you knew what we know about the most popular prescription and over-the-counter drugs, you'd be sick. That's why Dr. Douglass wrote this shocking report about the poisons in your medicine chest. He gives you the low-down on different categories of drugs. Everything from painkillers and cold remedies to tranquilizers and powerful cancer drugs.

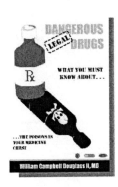

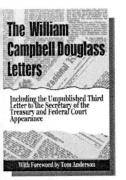

The William Campbell Douglass Letters.
Expose of Government Machinations
(Vietnam War).

THE WILLIAM CAMPBELL DOUGLASS LETTERS. Dr. Douglass' Defense in 1968 Tax Case and Expose of Government Machinations during the Vietnam War.

The Eagle's Feather. A Novel of
International Political Intrigue.

Although The Eagle's Feather is a work of fiction set in the 1970's, it is built, as with most fiction, on a framework of plausibility and background information. This is a fiction book that could not have been written were it not for various ominous aspects, which pose a clear and present danger to the security of the United States.

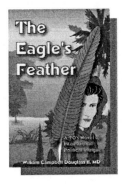

Rhino Publishing

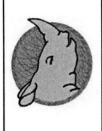

ORDER FORM

PURCHASER INFORMATION

Purchaser's Name (Please Print): _____

Shipping Address (Do not use a P.O. Box): _____

City: _____ State/Prov.: _____ Country: _____

Zip/Postal Code: _____ Telephone No.: _____ Fax No.: _____

E-Mail Address (if interested in receiving free e-Books when available): _____

CREDIT CARD INFO (CIRCLE ONE):

MASTERCARD, VISA, AMERICAN EXPRESS, DISCOVER, JCB, DINER'S CLUB, CARTE BLANCHE.

Charge my Card -> Number #: _____ Exp.: _____

*Security Code: _____ * Required for all MasterCard, Visa and American Express purchases. For your security, we require that you enter your card's verification number. The verification number is also called a CCV number. This code is the 3 digits farthest right in the signature field on the back of your VISA/MC, or the 4 digits to the right on the front of your American Express card. Your credit card statement will show **a different name than Rhino Publishing** as the vendor.

WE DO NOT share your private information, we use 3ʳᵈ party credit card processing service to process your order only.

ADDITIONAL INFORMATION

If your shipping address is not the same as your credit card billing address, please indicate your card billing address here.

_____   Type of card: _____

Name on the card

Billing Address: _____

City: _____   State/Prov.: _____   Zip/Postal Code: _____

Fax a copy of this order to:
RHINO PUBLISHING, S.A.
1-888-317-6767 or International #: + 416-352-5126

To order by mail, send your payment by first class mail only to the following address. Please include a copy of this order form. Make your check or bank drafts (NO postal money order) payable to RHINO PUBLISHING, S.A. and mail to:

Rhino Publishing, S.A.
Attention: PTY 5048
P.O. Box 025724
Miami, FL.
USA 33102

Digital E-books also available online: www.rhinopublish.com

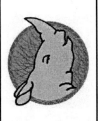

Rhino Publishing

ORDER
FORM

Purchaser's Name (Please Print):

I would like to order the following paperback book of Dr. Douglass (Alternative Medicine Books):

X	9962-636-04-3	Add 10 Years to Your Life. With some "best of" Dr. Douglass writings.	$13.99	$
X	9962-636-07-8	AIDS and Biological Warfare. What They Are Not Telling You!	$17.99	$
X	9962-636-09-4	Bad Medicine. How Individuals Get Killed By Bad Medicine.	$11.99	$
X	9962-636-10-8	Color Me Healthy. The Healing Power of Colors.	$11.99	$
X	9962-636 -XX-X	Color Filters for Color Me Healthy. 11 Basic Roscolene Filters for Lamps.	$21.89	$
X	9962-636-15-9	Dangerous Legal Drugs. The Poisons in Your Medicine Chest.	$13.99	$
X	9962-636-18-3	Dr. Douglass' Complete Guide to Better Vision. Improve eyesight naturally.	$11.99	$
X	9962-636-19-1	Eat Your Cholesterol! How to Live off the Fat of the Land and Feel Great.	$11.99	$
X	9962-636-12-4	Grandma Bell's A To Z Guide To Healing. Her Kitchen Cabinet Cures.	$14.99	$
X	9962-636-22-1	Hormone Replacement Therapies. Astonishing Results For Men & Women	$11.99	$
X	9962-636-25-6	Hydrogen Peroxide: One of the Most Underused Medical Miracle.	$15.99	$
X	9962-636-27-2	Into the Light. New Edition with Blood Irradiation Instrument Instructions.	$19.99	$
X	9962-636-54-X	Milk Book. The Classic on the Nutrition of Milk and How to Benefit from it.	$17.99	$

___ X	9962-636-00-0	Painful Dilemma - Patients in Pain - People in Prison.	$17.99 $ ___
___ X	9962-636-32-9	Prostate Problems. Safe, Simple, Effective Relief for Men over 50.	$11.99 $ ___
___ X	9962-636-34-5	St. Petersburg Nights. Enlightening Story of Life and Science in Russia.	$17.99 $ ___
___ X	9962-636-37-X	Stop Aging or Slow the Process. Exercise With Oxygen Therapy Can Help.	$11.99 $ ___
___ X	9962-636-60-4	The Hypertension Report. Say Good Bye to High Blood Pressure.	$11.99 $ ___
___ X	9962-636-48-5	The Joy of Mature Sex and How to Be a Better Lover...	$13.99 $ ___
___ X	9962-636-43-4	The Smoker's Paradox: Health Benefits of Tobacco.	$14.99 $ ___

Political Books:

___ X	9962-636-40-X	The Eagle's Feather. A 70's Novel of International Political Intrigue.	$15.99 $ ___
___ X	9962-636-46-9	The W. C. D. Letters. Expose of Government Machinations (Vietnam War).	$11.99 $ ___

SUB-TOTAL: $ ___

ADD $5.00 HANDLING FOR YOUR ORDER: $ 5.00 $ 5.00

___ X ADD $2.50 SHIPPING FOR EACH ITEM ON ORDER: $ 2.50 $ ___

NOTE THAT THE MINIMUM SHIPPING AND HANDLING IS $7.50 FOR 1 BOOK ($5.00 + $2.50)

For order shipped outside the US, add $5.00 per item

___ X ADD $5.00 S. & H. OR EACH ITEM ON ORDER (INTERNATIONAL ORDERS ONLY) $ 5.00 $ ___

Allow up to 21 days for delivery (we will call you about back orders if any)

TOTAL: $ ___

Fax a copy of this order to: 1-888-317-6767 or Int'l + 416-352-5126
or mail to: Rhino Publishing, S.A. Attention: PTY 5048 P.O. Box 025724, Miami, FL., 33102 USA
Digital E-books also available online: www.rhinopublish.com